THE GUIDE TO MODERN
CUPPING THERAPY

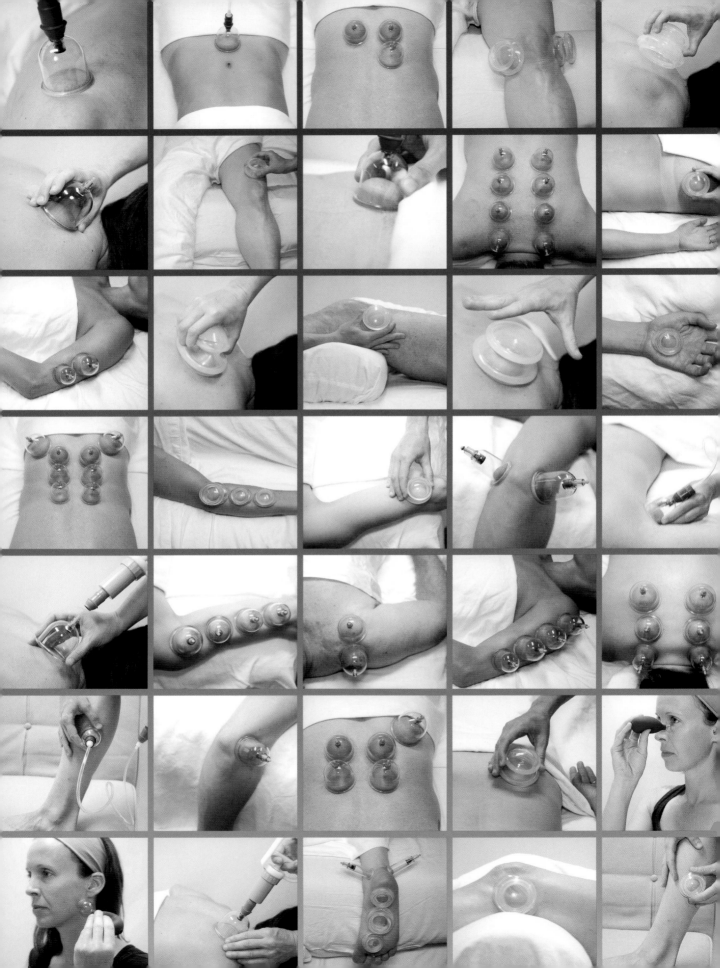

THE GUIDE TO MODERN CUPPING THERAPY

Your Step-by-Step Source for Vacuum Therapy

Shannon Gilmartin, CMT

Robert
ROSE

For complete cataloguing information, see page 251.

Disclaimer

This book is a general guide only and should never be a substitute for the skill,
knowledge, and experience of a qualified medical professional dealing with the facts,
circumstances, and symptoms of a particular case.

The nutritional, medical, and health information presented in this book is based
on the research, training, and professional experience of the author, and is true
and complete to the best of her knowledge. However, this book is intended only
as an informative guide for those wishing to know more about health, nutrition,
and medicine; it is not intended to replace or countermand the advice given by the
reader's personal physician. Because each person and situation is unique, the author
and the publisher urge the reader to check with a qualified health-care professional
before using any procedure where there is a question as to its appropriateness. A
physician should be consulted before beginning any exercise program. The author
and the publisher are not responsible for any adverse effects or consequences
resulting from the use of the information in this book. It is the responsibility of the
reader to consult a physician or other qualified health-care professional regarding his
or her personal care.

Editor: Fina Scroppo
Copyeditor: Sheila Wawanash
Indexer: Belle Wong
Design and Production: PageWave Graphics Inc.
Photography: Jennifer Steele (except as noted below)
Illustrations: Kveta (except as noted below)

Additional photographs: pages 11, 71 and 123 © gettyimages.com; page 12 ©
Wellcome Library, London. Wellcome Images images@wellcome.ac.uk; page 13 ©
Steve F-E-Cameron (page 12); page 19 (top left) Robert Stern. Used with permission
from Global Healthworks Foundation; page 19 (remainder) Malike Sibide. Used with
permission from Global Healthworks Foundation.; select images on pages 80, 81,
248, 249 by Shannon Gilmartin.

Additional illustrations: page 35 Alicia McCarthy/PageWave Graphics Inc.; pages 178
and 184 © gettyimages.ca.

Published by Robert Rose Inc.
120 Eglinton Avenue East, Suite 800, Toronto, Ontario, Canada M4P 1E2
Tel: (416) 322-6552 Fax: (416) 322-6936
www.robertrose.ca

Printed and bound in Canada

2 3 4 5 6 7 8 9 TCP 25 24 23 22 21 20 19 18

CONTENTS

PART 3
TREATING COMMON CONDITIONS WITH CUPPING

CHAPTER 8: BASIC APPLICATIONS FOR COMMON CONDITIONS: THERAPIST AND SELF-CARE OPTIONS

Introduction

I LOVE CUPS. These wonderful tools have truly been the greatest addition to my professional practice and have been exceptionally rewarding in my own life.

As a bodyworker, the results from cupping have been extraordinary year after year and client after client. I've seen results, from subtle to miraculous, and I am continuously humbled by the power of therapeutic cupping.

As a teacher, I thoroughly enjoy sharing this amazing modality of healing bodywork with the countless students I have had the privilege to teach. There is nothing like watching people learn, assimilate and be thoroughly inspired by the information associated with this alternative therapy.

As a recipient, therapeutic cups have changed my life. From reducing the appearance of a large scar on my face and relieving chronic pain to enhancing my own athletic performance, I have personally experienced the rewarding results and I am proud to be a walking testimonial to this incredible therapy.

Thus I am writing this book after many years of experience with regular, clinical applications of therapeutic cupping infused with my own methods of therapeutic bodywork, as well as after teaching in many parts of the world, including the United States, Canada, Guatemala, Ireland and Italy.

Many diverse therapeutic cupping techniques have been employed by health-care workers and caretakers of every ethnicity for thousands of years, from bleeding cups that literally remove unwanted blood from the body to cups that are used to dispel energy stagnations or relieve muscle pain. Although it is an ancient practice, the efficacy of cupping has been under a shroud of mystery for a long time, with no clear indications of how cupping affects the human body and why it is so therapeutically successful. Recently, this wonderful modality has found its way into modern bodywork practices. From massage therapists, physical therapists and estheticians to sports trainers, chiropractors and doctors (whether doctors are using cups in their own practices or referring patients to a bodyworker who uses cups), it seems everyone knows someone who knows something about cupping! In recent years, there has also been a broader awareness and interest in cupping as the world saw Olympic athletes displaying cupping marks with great pride, as well as various celebrities acknowledge a fondness for cupping. Its "secrets" remain untold, however, so I've written this book hoping to uncover the many mysteries and clarify the techniques that surround this unique therapy and its wonderful tools.

I have been actively using cupping since 2004 in my own therapeutic bodywork practice, and the results have been truly awe-inspiring. For the many clients I have treated with cupping — among them those who have experienced either chronic pain, acute injuries, post-surgical (or post-accident) rehabilitation, inflammatory pathologies, stressful conditions or reduced athletic performance — cups seem like the best tool as an adjunct for all kinds of relief, yet this therapy is constantly being discovered.

I have worked with cups in quite different environments and interesting applications, but the general guidelines have always emphasized safe, logical and therapeutic usage. Like many practices, you may have come across some dangerous and downright weird applications online, but cupping isn't as simple as "place a cup here and feel better." A high degree of safety and skillful technique is involved in the proper application of cups.

The use of cups in a therapeutic manner is truly an art form open to the user's interpretation. Applications of cupping can be altered to fit the needs of the person applying them — whether using cups to relax someone or to address muscular tension or even breathing restrictions, a certain skillset of working on the human body, along with creativity, is key. Even with this freedom of variation, however, there should be a uniform rule of safety first and foremost.

The Guide to Modern Cupping Therapy is designed to appeal as much to the professional bodyworker as it is to those who have an interest in therapeutic cupping for their own use. Over 10 concise chapters, readers can expect a thorough review of the technique and its applications, including step-by-step basic and alternative applications to treat some of the most common physical discomforts and health conditions.

There have been far more questions than answers when it comes to cupping…until now. *For the professional bodyworker*, this book offers:

- Step-by-step guidance in using cups safely and effectively as part of an existing treatment plan
- Scientific information on the effects of therapeutic cupping on the human body
- Education on the marks and tissue responses to this work
- Proper applications to ensure cups are used to their greatest potential, depending on how they are incorporated into a clinician's own body of work
- Information on safe and effective, non-bruising applications to ensure you are getting the best results possible without causing harm (No bodyworker should ever tell their clients that bruising is good for them.)

For the non-professional bodyworker, this book is equally beneficial, providing the science, education, safety, step-by-step application and guidelines so you can use cupping on a loved one or administer the therapy on your own body. This book also includes some education on the composition and functioning of the human body, especially with regard to how cupping can affect these body systems (see Chapter 3). While at times the anatomical information may seem overly specific, a thorough grounding in this subject is really contained in these details — right down to cellular functioning.

I always encourage those who are interested in learning more about the cup's true potential to attend a live workshop; however, I can confidently say that this book will give them a useful introduction and understanding of when and how cupping can be used, as well as the extraordinary results it can achieve.

PART 1
CUPPING ON THE BODY

CHAPTER 1

The History of Cupping and Vacuum Therapies

CUPPING IN WORLD HISTORY

CUPPING 101

Humans have an inherent instinct for vacuum therapy by the use of oral suction. People try to suck out a wooden splinter or poisonous venom, or employ suction as an immediate reaction to injury; for example, when you hurt your finger.

Cupping has been used for thousands of years. Different cultures have used cups, along with the negative pressure created inside them, in their own unique way, primarily to remove, or "suction," unwanted materials from the body, whether to draw out sickness, pains, pathogenic substances or evil spirits. Today, bodywork practitioners have steadily adopted cupping as a complementary and alternative therapy to treat everything from constipation to cellulite to back and shoulder pain.

Historical Methods of Cupping

Throughout history, there have been two primary methods of applied suction, or "vacuum," therapy with cups: dry cupping (suction is placed directly on the skin) and wet cupping (the skin is cut to physically draw out any unwanted or stagnant substances, such as blood, poison, venom, pus). Dry cupping, the more familiar method of application, requires no cutting and will be the focus of this book.

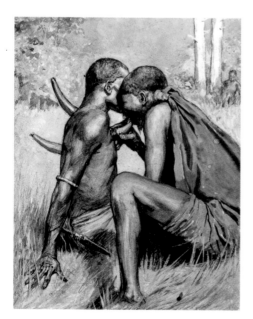

Primitive Cups

Over the centuries, cups have been made around the world from animal horns, bamboo, clay, metal and glass. Some of the most primitive methods of suction therapy have featured hollowed-out animal horns that were applied to specific points on the body by a medicine person, who would use oral suction to draw out toxins, such as venom from snakebites, or drain blood or pus from skin boils. Later, to prevent the medicine person from ingesting harmful material, chewed-up grass or other organic materials were inserted into the hollowed horn to obstruct airflow and create suction pressure as the air was being sucked out. Suction methods eventually progressed to include the use of fire, where the burning of materials such as cotton would consume the enclosed air, creating a vacuum within a cupping vessel.

Ancient Egypt

In Ancient Egypt, Imhotep, who was known as the first physician and the god of medicine, advocated for the practice of cupping. Hieroglyphics of that time (shown below) depict cups as medical instruments, along with knives, hooks and forceps. Cupping was part of the practice of medicine: records in the ancient medical texts of the Ebers Papyrus (circa 1550 BCE) describe the use of cups to treat vertigo, pain, appetite imbalances, menstruation problems and other ailments — ultimately encouraging a "healing crisis" in the body.

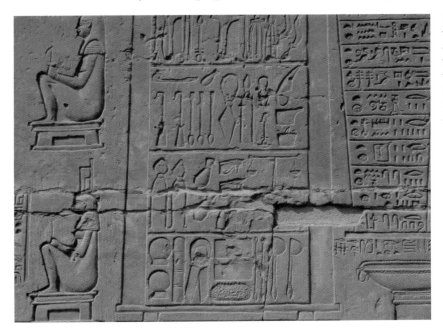

Images of hieroglyphics from the walls of the double temple of Kom Ombo, dedicated to Sobek and Horus, depict various medical instruments in use at the time, including knives, saws, hooks, forceps and cupping vessels.

Ancient Greece

From Egypt, cupping made its way into Greek medical practices. Hippocrates, the father of modern medicine, studied at the temple of Imhotep along with other Greek physicians and adopted the use of cupping, among other medical practices. Hippocrates designated methods of care to address the body's vital elements of health, the four humors — blood, phlegm, yellow bile and black bile. He surmised that if all the humors are in balance, then the body is healthy. An excess or lack of any humor can create disease and dysfunction, however, so he created specific treatments. Ancient Greek Unani medicine used both wet and dry cupping to promote balance among the humors.

Hippocrates used many cupping applications for healing the body, including treatment for musculoskeletal pains, illnesses or dysfunctions related to the head, torso and gynecological region. After Hippocrates, the Greek physician Galen continued the advocacy of cupping therapy and prescribed it regularly. Others followed in the footsteps of such great physicians. In 413 BCE, Herodotus, a physician and historian, wrote:

"Scarification with Cupping possesses the power of evacuating offending matter from the head; of diminishing pain of the same part; of lessening inflammation; of restoring the appetite; of strengthening a weak stomach; of removing vertigo and a tendency to faint; of drawing deep-seated offending matter towards the surface; of drying up fluxions; checking hemorrhages; promoting menstrual evacuations; arresting the tendency to putrefaction in fevers; allaying rigors; accelerating and moderating the crisis of diseases; removing a propensity to somnolence; conciliating natural repose; removing heaviness. These, and many analogous maladies, are relieved by the judicious application of the Cucurbits (Cups), dry or bloody."

In ancient Greek Hippocratic practices, physicians referred to cupping as *sikia* or *vendouzes*, a term and practice still used today. Ask any Greek person and they'll likely tell you about a family member who performs a version of cure-all cupping — typically stationary cups or "flash" cupping — to remedy a cough, cold, fever or body ache. Traditional Greek homes often have some small glass jars, even empty baby food jars, and cotton to light and suck the air out of the cup, ready to use for quick home cupping. Practices like this are as common as the modern-day convention of keeping an ice pack handy as a first-aid remedy for injuries or of keeping over-the-counter pain relief in the medicine cabinet.

Islamic Practice

In Islamic medicine, therapeutic cupping is called *hijama*, or "drawing out," from the root word *al-hajm*, or "sucking." Over the centuries, the applications of cups have been incredibly diverse and were used for everything from expelling evil spirits to treating muscle aches to stress relief. It was often referred to as one of the most powerful methods of healing, noted for moving vital life energy within the blood (comparable to *qi*, or *chi*, in Chinese medicine), along with the removal of toxins and waste materials from the blood. Cupping was said to be the best method to either recover from ailments or prevent disease. In historical texts, there were references to the best days to apply cupping, stories of angels instructing Mohammed to use cups and to the use of cupping on individuals afflicted in some way.

Chinese Medicine

For thousands of years, Chinese culture has probably been most closely associated with cupping therapy, more specifically among acupuncturists and Traditional Chinese Medicine (TCM) practitioners.

One of the earliest records of cupping therapy was found in the Mawangdui Silk Texts, or *boshu*, ancient medical texts that were

---

written on silks and discovered in a tomb from the Han Dynasty. There are many examples of cupping therapies in one of the world's oldest medical textbooks, *Huang Di Nei Jing* — *The Yellow Emperor's Classic of Medicine*. A famous alchemist and herbalist, Ge Hong (283–343 CE) popularized the saying, "Acupuncture and cupping, more than half of the ills cured."

Cupping is a common modality of healing within Traditional Chinese Medicine. TCM practitioners use therapies such as acupuncture with needles, moxibustion, gua sha (scraping) and cupping to remove any stagnations of invasive pathogens — wind, cold, heat or dampness — that could alter the life energy in the body, known as *qi* or *chi*. Such interruptions in the flow of *qi* and blood can alter a person's wellness, which may result in a loss of function, or sensation, pain and possibly disease.

Cups are applied to any area that interrupts this flow of energy — within channels of energy — to purge these materials from the body. Cupping facilitates the return of the body's energies to a natural fluidity and restores full function, normal sensation, comfort and the balance of health.

The markings, or *sha* ("toxins"), that result from scraping or cupping techniques represent the release of these invasive materials. After multiple treatments, the intensity of their color will typically lessen, indicating the progressive removal of such materials from the body. It has been thought that the darker the colors, the deeper or more severe the stagnation. When interviewed about various cupping marks, Susan Sandage, a licensed acupuncturist and diplomate of Oriental medicine (as per the National Certification Commission for Acupuncture and Oriental Medicine, or NCCAOM), described the tissue response to a cold pathogen as similar to other cupping markings: when a cold pathogen has been discovered, one may see a blanched, dusky area appearing on the skin, or the area may be cold to the touch. When this cold pathogen has been released from the body, the area will no longer present blanched tissue or feel cold to the touch.

Europe

Cupping is used extensively throughout East and West Europe, and it is not difficult to find descendants of Europeans sharing stories of their ancestors using the modality. Similar methods of cupping, such as stationary cups to treat sickness and muscle aches, have been used throughout Europe over the centuries and continue to be used into modern times. In Germany, cupping therapy is known as *schröpfkopfbehandlung* or simply *schröpfen;* in Poland and Bulgaria, cupping has been used since the 19th century for various healing practices; and in Italy, many are familiar with the use of in-home cup therapy for coughs and colds as well as muscular aches and pains.

A client's personal story of cupping use in a traditional Italian home:

My grandmother and then my mother would cup us when we had aches. They would use cotton pieces, wrap them around a coin and form a sort of a wick on top, and then place it on the skin wherever the muscle ache was. They would then ignite the wick and place an inverted glass over it, and when it would smoke inside the cup, the skin would puff up where the muscles ached. While some might have believed such a practice was superstitious, the area would not puff up if there was nothing to be released. Once they finished, the ache would be gone. ~ M.M.

The Americas

Cups have a rich history in the North, Central and Southern Americas, too. Native American medicine women were known to employ cups as a healing modality. Cups were used to treat physical ailments like pain, swelling or rheumatism, but also to expel negative spiritual energies. Most common cups used were hollowed animal horns as the suction vessel, and the cupping was mostly for bloodletting, or wet cupping.

As early as the 1700s, American doctors were using cupping regularly in their medical practices and medical suppliers were carrying cupping sets in their standard inventory. When doctors made house calls, they often carried cupping instruments in their bags.

The 19th Century

The 1800s brought both progress and a growing skepticism about cupping in the medical communities. Many health-care professionals advocated for its use, including practitioners like well-known British cupper Samuel Bayfield, who described cupping as an art and its benefits as far-reaching. In 1826, a surgeon named Charles Kennedy said, "The art of Cupping has been so well known, and the benefits arising from it so long experienced, that it is quite unnecessary to bring forward testimonials in favour of what has received not only the approbation of modern times, but also the sanction of the remotest antiquity." Nevertheless, there were skeptics who questioned its efficacy.

Later in the century, the use of cupping was questioned by doctors who practiced Western, or modern, medicine. Their practices focused on addressing internal ailments, including the introduction of pharmaceutical medications, rather than treating the body from the outside in, and these practitioners began seeking scientific support for the therapeutic benefits of cupping. Since its efficacy could not be proven by modern scientific measures, the effectiveness of cupping came into question and its decline began.

CONTEMPORARY CUPPING TECHNIQUES

Modern Use

While the practice of cupping dwindled among Western practitioners, it still had a thriving existence in other societies. In 1946, British author George Orwell's essay "How the Poor Die" made reference to cupping for treating pneumonia while he was in a hospital in Paris, France. The Russian Ministry of Health has done more than 40 years of clinical research on cupping therapies, and in the 1950s, both Chinese and Russian hospitals established the use of such therapies to treat patients in their facilities. The British Cupping Society (BCS) was formed in England in 2008 and many international health ministries now use it as the benchmark for ethical practices, education and standards in the field of cupping therapies.

In more recent years, therapeutic cupping has experienced an interesting resurgence and become a tool that crosses over all professional areas of therapeutic bodywork. Not only do acupuncturists and Traditional Chinese Medicine practitioners still use cups, but so too do massage therapists, physical therapists, athletic trainers and other bodyworkers.

In the 1980s and '90s, cupping had a sort of renaissance within the medical community, both in traditional and alternative practices. Modern practitioners like Bruce Bentley and Ilkay Chirali, who are both well regarded in the field of modern Eastern and Western applications of cupping therapies, have been prominent advocates for this work. Alternative applications have also continued to grow in popularity, such as the work of Anita Shannon, a cosmetologist and massage therapist who has implemented modified versions of cupping into her bodywork practices with gentler, less invasive applications alongside the more traditional cupping techniques.

Massage and Therapeutic Bodywork

The growing interest in cupping therapies has brought a surge of varied styles to fit the demands of a more broad-spectrum, diverse world of bodywork. The variety of applications and lack of regulation, however, have resulted in instances of harmful and dangerous cupping work. Cupping marks, for example, are often incorrectly referred to as "bruises," and while most cupping therapies used around the world should never bruise (or hurt), bodyworkers who use cups without proper training may potentially bruise an individual if they're operating with the wrong intent that "stronger suction is better" or if they inform clients that "the bruise is good for you." Bruises are never helpful and a stronger suction is not always better.

DID YOU KNOW?

The dynamic potential of vacuum therapies continues to grow, with more and more therapy centers offering cupping as a service and teaching techniques to student practitioners.

However, many of today's therapeutic bodywork practitioners, including massage and physical therapists, sports trainers and chiropractors, use cupping in a variety of safe and effective ways that complement their own professional modalities to help loosen muscles, increase flexibility and facilitate manipulations, among other applications.

Adaptations of Cupping Therapy

- **Cellulite treatment in spas:** Day spas have been using vacuum devices to treat cellulite for years. These facilities usually own mechanical suction devices that use pressure and various applications, such as vibrations and pumping, to target areas with cellulite.
- **The breast pump:** Used as a means of collecting breast milk, or when lactation dysfunction occurs, such a device can soften the breast tissue and encourage the flow of milk. The same devices have been used to treat other conditions associated with breast tissue, such as plugged milk ducts or even mastectomy reconstruction procedures — applications that should be administered by licensed professional bodyworkers trained to do so.
- **The penis pump:** In addition to drawing fluid into the tissue to encourage growth, the penis pump can also be used to treat Peyronie's disease, a scarring of the penile structure, most likely due to previous trauma or breakage.
- **First-aid venom extraction kits (with small sets of cups):** These cups are meant to pull toxins out of the body when treating beestings and snakebites. You can find these tiny cups and vacuum plungers in most pharmacies.

Universal Applications

From the most ancient civilizations to modern clinical applications of vacuum therapies, cupping has become a universal therapeutic tool. In the next several chapters, you will learn how to apply cupping applications that have transitioned from past uses to modern-day practices.

- While Chinese practitioners addressed the circulation of *qi*, you will learn about the therapeutic effects of encouraging the circulation of blood and lymph in the body.
- While some cultures have addressed stagnation of various invasive pathogens, you will learn how to address stagnation of various materials in the body, such as injured muscle tissue, inflammation and lymph.
- While some civilizations have used cups to expel "evil" spirits you will learn how cups can be used to relieve stress.

Client Work

With the Global Healthworks Foundation, I had the good fortune of working with some local health promoters in rural communities in Guatemala. While teaching them how to use the cups, I would often see them smiling comfortably at me, since their Mayan ancestors had been using *copitas* for generations.

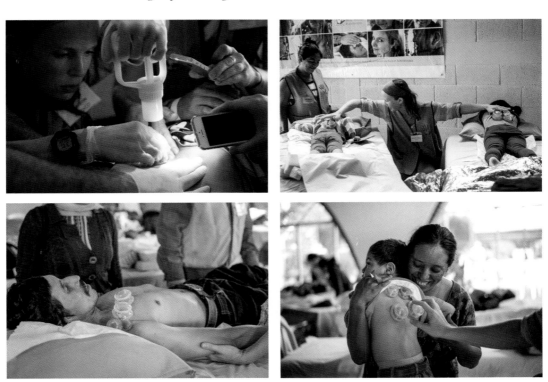

CHAPTER 2

How Cupping Affects the Body

PHYSIOLOGICAL RESPONSES

Understanding how cups work on a physiological level offers some insight into why cups have been used for overall wellness throughout recorded history. Each body system will have a different reaction to cupping (more on that in the next chapter), but there are also a few basic mechanisms that occur when cups are applied to the body.

The primary mechanisms include:

Note

Unless stated otherwise, references to "pressure" will mean the negative pressure from applied suction.

1. Negative pressure
2. Vasodilation
3. Enhanced fluid exchange

Keep these three physiological responses in mind as we progress into a deeper understanding of why cupping is so effective.

Negative Pressure

Once applied, cups lift the tissue and begin to take effect with negative pressure. This pressure creates a pulling action, which allows for the separation of fused or adhered tissue.

The body strives for fluidity and suppleness — inside and out — to provide the best environment possible for optimal bodily functions. Any tissue that is "stuck" inhibits optimal functioning. Whether tissues are stuck as the result of dehydration, chronic inflammation, repetitive motion injuries (when muscles can stick together from fascial binding) or any other cause, tissues that are adhered are not in their ideal condition.

This same pulling action can draw out any interstitial debris (see page 22) that may be trapped within the soft tissues.

Anatomy FYI

An *adhesion* is any two anatomical surfaces stuck or growing together that do not naturally connect, usually due to injury or inflammation. The iliotibial (IT) band along the thigh can develop adhesions whenever it becomes extraordinarily tight; for example, after a long run.

The human anatomy has an impressive capacity to store material within the layers of tissue. The body primarily focuses on remaining an intact, single unit contained within the outer protective layer of the skin. Connective tissues are meant to do exactly what their name implies — keep the body connected; that is, ensure that everything is attached where it should be for optimal functioning. Anything that tries to interrupt this harmonious balance may become tangled in the fibers of various tissues as the body struggles to maintain its structural integrity around this unwanted material. Cupping can work to draw such materials out. A simple comparison is to what a household vacuum does for carpets — cups can do the same for the body.

Vasodilation

Vasodilation is the action of widening blood vessels and is usually activated by the relaxation of smooth muscle tissue in any given area. Cups stimulate a local response within the underlying tissue structures, promoting the release of vaso-activating chemicals, such as histamines, which in turn encourages the lumen (see Anatomy FYI, below) of the blood vessels to dilate. A similar response is achieved by massage or applying either heat or prolonged cold applications. This vascular dilation allows for fluids to rush into or *through* an area.

Anatomy FYI

A *lumen* is any opening channel where materials pass through a tube. Blood passes through the lumen of a blood vessel. Food passes through the lumen of the large intestine before exiting the body.

Enhanced Fluid Exchange

Cupping has a powerful effect on blood, interstitial fluids (those that surround cells) and lymph. Cups act as a vacuum, drawing fluids into an area or encouraging them through their respective exchange processes. The capillaries host various fluid-exchanging processes (diffusion, filtration, osmosis and active transport). These processes allow nutrient-rich fluids to feed cells while removing waste material at the same time. The vacuum effect of cupping pulls blood into dehydrated, malnourished or ischemic (deficient in blood) tissues. Due to their suction pump effect on the body, cups also encourage venous return and lymph fluid movements.

The combination of negative pressure, vasodilation and enhanced fluid exchange allows for some incredible reactions to take place within the body. But before we go further, it is important to understand how the presence of adhesions and interstitial debris can adversely affect the human body.

What is an Adhesion?

Adhesions are defined as any two anatomical surfaces stuck or growing together that do not naturally connect, usually due to injury or inflammation. This can be within muscles, connective tissues (like fascia), visceral organs and across body systems (for example, parts of the dermis adhering to muscles wherever fascia may be tight and restricted).

At any level of anatomy, an adhesion obstructs optimal bodily functions; whether inhibiting the circulation of bodily fluids, impairing muscular activities or interfering with systemic activities (for example, normal bowel movements). Human anatomy is organized in its form to function without interruption, and adhesions alter this harmonious balance and structural order, which can lead to dysfunction.

What is Interstitial Debris?

Interstitial debris is any material that the body could not dispose of on its own. This material can include:

- Old blood deposits from injury or surgeries
- Cellular waste that the lymphatic system could not assimilate (see Chapter 3: "Therapeutic Benefits on the Body Systems" for more information about lymph)
- Metabolic waste (e.g., lactic acid)
- Medications
- Toxins (e.g., chemical exposures)
- Foreign objects (e.g., stitches, pieces of glass from a motor vehicle accident, etc.)

While some materials, such as old blood, may seem like they wouldn't cause any real harm if they're not removed, consider this example.

> When a pebble is dropped into a tranquil pond, it disturbs the entire body of water. The pebble then settles below the surface and sits at the bottom of the pond. Water will maneuver around, making space for the pebble to the best of its ability. The pebble will remain at the bottom until it's forcefully removed. Naturally, the water will not push the pebble to the surface.
>
> Now picture the pebble as interstitial debris and the pond as our body. The bottom of the pond is the layers of tissue where interstitial debris may reside.

The Body's Response

When our bodies encounter interstitial debris, a number of reactions take place, including the following:

- The body makes a serious effort to maintain overall well-being, and to do so, it requires a smooth-moving, fluid environment (blood, lymph, soft tissues, natural bodily functions). The "speed bump" of interstitial debris is now ruining this flow.

- The body tries naturally to expel any variety of interstitial debris, but this can prove to be an arduous task. While the body tries to push out these materials, the connective tissues attempt to maintain their structural integrity as a priority, which inevitably overpowers the act of expulsion.
- Restriction wins and a vicious cycle of ineffective waste removal begins.

Here's another way to look at it. Say you were lifting a heavy object and you created microtears, or tiny tears in the tight muscle fibers of the muscles being used. Various blood vessels that innervate these muscles struggle through the layers of muscle fibers to push the tissue debris out to the surface, where the lymphatic system can dispose of it. Once the waste is gone, healthy blood can be pumped in to replace the waste, fill the space it previously occupied and heal the area. This capability is challenged, however, because the tissue is too tight — perhaps due to the presence of adhesions within the muscle tissue — to allow this healing process to flow properly. The waste in the torn muscle tissue remains, creating a stagnation that the body cannot fully express into the lymphatic system and the ripple effect begins to take hold. Fluids get backed up and displaced (edema), muscles are not properly supplied with blood (ischemia), perhaps the inflammatory material that was sent to heal the area cannot function fully and gets trapped (embedded inflammation), full engagement of muscle function is hindered (dysfunction) and the overall health of the muscle is now impaired.

Persistent interstitial debris leads to a ripple effect of varying proportions. The body can literally bury these materials within itself and try to operate around it. These obstacles — whether they are accumulated blood cells in an injured muscle or glass that wasn't removed properly after an accident — alter the body's optimal functioning patterns and can lead to a whole slew of dysfunctions.

Cupping is beneficial because it promotes suppleness within soft tissues and facilitates the body's desire to get rid of waste, which it sometimes simply cannot do completely on its own.

CUPPING 101

Cups can affect tissue as far as 4 inches (10 cm) into the human body.

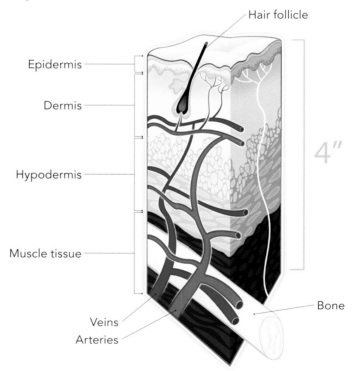

Hair follicle

Epidermis

Dermis

Hypodermis

Muscle tissue

4"

Bone

Veins

Arteries

Other Ways Cupping Can Benefit the Entire Body

- **Cups encourage circulation.** One of cupping's impressive benefits is how the therapy stimulates overall circulation, even down to the capillary level (microcirculation). Skin, muscles and visceral organs all respond positively to the promotion of this delicate process.

- **Cups alleviate adhesions.** Another extraordinary benefit offered by cupping is how it addresses adhesions. The ability to lift and separate tissue while simultaneously offering hydration to that which was previously restricted is incredibly therapeutic.

- **Cups help clear congestion and stagnation.** Anything that is stagnant in an otherwise healthy internal environment is what predominantly leads to dysfunction and disease. Cups help clear stagnation from skin, muscles, bones, joints, organs and even energies (whether emotional energies that lead to physical manifestations or energies relating to vital life forces, like Traditional Chinese Medicine that uses cups to influence *qi*) — everything! For example, limited movement of a joint (such as frozen shoulder) can be caused by a stagnation of inflammatory materials. This trapped heat (inflammation) can dehydrate the surrounding muscles, leading to a lack of flexibility, which ultimately progresses to limited range of motion. (See Chapter 8 for applications to treat frozen shoulder, page 149.)

  Another example is cellulite. Challenged circulation in the hips and gluteal region can lead to a stagnation of lymph fluids, which cannot maneuver around the congested adipose tissue that is stuck between the micro-adhesions of connective tissue (See Chapter 10 for more details on working with cellulite.) Cups enable optimal fluidity to return to the body.

- **Cups can lift, rehydrate and manipulate fascia.** Fascia is a form of connective tissue that envelops all muscle tissues, is interwoven throughout all structures of anatomy, and contributes to maintaining structural integrity of the entire human body. Fascial restrictions can be challenging to release in therapies like massage or physical rehabilitation, so working with cups can help facilitate some impressive results. Cupping forces hydration to pass through these fluid-rich structures, which can improve pliability to what may have been otherwise dehydrated and therefore adhered structures. The negative pressure allows for a lifting and stretching mechanism to occur, and this provides an opportunity to create space where it was lacking. All of this allows for a potentially substantial change in otherwise restricted or immobilized areas.

DID YOU KNOW?

Environmental factors like diet and exercise, as well as unhealthy habits such as smoking, can alter an optimal state of well-being. Physical manifestations of these factors can include dehydration, limited range of motion, stiffness or constipation.

- **Cups can cause microtrauma in tissues.** Although this response sounds counterproductive, cupping can bring about beneficial inflammation to encourage deep-seated restrictions to clear and rebuild healthy tissue, thus encouraging the body's own process of regeneration. This is why it is so important to apply appropriate suction. An increase to a stronger suction is only recommended when the person's body is receptive to it — meaning no pain or discomfort is felt when cups are applied, rather than immediately applying suction that is potentially too strong and causing damage.

Safety Point

It is important to acknowledge that while these microtraumas are beneficial, cupping that is too strong can cause damaging trauma and contusions. See Chapter 5: "Safe Cupping," as well as "Working with Inflammation" in Chapter 10 for more information.

- **Cups encourage neovascularization.** Neovascularization is the process by which new blood vessels form from already existing healthy vessels, bringing a fresh supply of nutrients and oxygen to previously deficient tissues. In areas of injury or damaged tissue (for example, excessive physical exertion leading to muscle tearing), cupping can stimulate this response in regional tissues, which in turn can speed recovery. Again, do not use cupping directly on severely injured tissue.
- **Cups help alleviate excessive pressure on sensory organs in soft tissue, which leads to a reduction in pain.** When soft tissue is restricted, it can cause the nerve endings that respond to pain to become overactive, stuck in a state of pain alert. The vasodilation response, along with the applied negative pressure, encourages these tight tissues to relax, thereby releasing the tension on the sensory organs involved.

Anatomy FYI

Nerve endings are part of the peripheral nervous system and are located throughout the body — skin, muscles, organs and connective tissues. See Chapter 3: "Therapeutic Benefits on the Body Systems," for more information.

Hydration

Cupping therapies generate a continuous movement of fluids within the layers of soft tissue. This concept is imperative to grasp. For cups to pull fluids into all the layers of tissue, these fluids must come from somewhere. Cupping brings about a continuous process of drawing fluids from surrounding cell spaces, from general circulation and from deeper layers of more hydrated tissues. Cupping therapies essentially leave people internally dehydrated.

The internal environment of our bodies requires a lot of water to survive. Have you ever experienced a headache and later discovered that you were dehydrated? The brain requires a lot of water, and it will pull from every available space (cells, intercellular) to access water reserves to perform its functions properly. Have you ever had a headache dissipate after drinking some water or water with electrolytes? Every internal organ demands water to function, and since cupping pulls water to the surface tissues, it is important to replenish the never–ending internal demand, to maintain all-around wellness. The skin, the surface layer where cups are attached, can also become dehydrated.

The tissues being cupped are being hydrated from the inside out. It is imperative to replenish the internal source by drinking water. While there may be various schools of thought on how much water to drink, the majority agree that you need to drink a significant quantity of water every day, especially when receiving cupping therapies.

Effects of Dehydration After Cupping

If water is insufficiently replenished, the entire body can suffer. Not only is the removal of toxins and waste materials (for example, lactic acid) inhibited — which can contribute to a less–than–great feeling after any cupping treatment — but muscles can cramp during or after treatment, too. The person may also experience an overall feeling of discomfort, such as headaches or even nausea. If the body is dehydrated when cupping is applied, it will try to gather the water by pulling it from any area possible (even pulling blood from muscle tissue), which can lead to a deficiency, such as muscle cramps, if it is not replenished. Just the same, it's best to rely on old-fashioned hydration by drinking water. One of the greatest complements to any cupping therapy is to drink plenty of water before *and* after treatment sessions.

DID YOU KNOW?

One way to measure how much water you should drink is by dividing your body weight (in pounds) in half and drinking that number in ounces. So, if you weigh 140 pounds you should drink 70 ounces of water a day. The old saying "8 to 10 glasses of water daily" should be considered an average daily minimum.

COMMON QUESTIONS ABOUT CUPPING

How do cups feel?

People have described the feeling of having cups applied to their body in many different ways. Examples range from feeling soft, soothing, rolling, invigorating, stimulating, energizing, penetrating, warming, tingling, ticklish and separating, to feeling like deep-tissue massage. People can feel itchy after cupping, most likely due to either an increase in circulation in the area (released histamines), the stimulation of nerve endings or the release of embedded inflammation.

Here's what some recipients have noted after treatment:

- "It feels like your hands but different."
- "It feels like I have breathing room in my tissues."
- "It sometimes feels like you found *the spot* no one has gotten to before with massage and bodywork!"

Even very strong suction should not hurt when done correctly. If the goal is to release deep muscular restrictions with strong stationary cups, be sure to start with lighter suction, increasing only when the body has adapted to this initial application and the recipient feels no discomfort. Never force suction, and respect the fact that sensitivity ranges dramatically from person to person. One of the most common mistakes is made when the person applying cups (whether to someone else or self-care) becomes overly zealous. While cups can yield some impressive and immediate results, attempting to "pull out the problem" in one application is not only dangerous but irrational — this work is *cumulative*.

Cupping works to unblock anything obstructing the continuous flow of life energies — bodily functions — within the body. Anything too aggressive or intense can harm this balance, or homeostasis. Cups should feel good; if they don't, the application should be adjusted until they do.

What are the marks that often happen from cupping?

Cupping marks are a sign of interstitial debris, such as old blood, being released after cups have been applied to the body. Cups work as a vacuum, helping to facilitate the release of any waste materials that the body sometimes simply cannot do on its own. While true cupping marks are a sign of release, sometimes bruises occur if this therapy is applied too strongly or too aggressively. For more information on these cupping marks, see Chapter 4: "Assessing the Skin after Treatment."

For how long can cups be applied? And how strong a suction can be used?

Everyone will experience a different reaction to therapeutic cupping. It is best, therefore, to limit both the time and the pressure of

Safety Point

Cupping can be a truly indescribable sensation, but no matter how someone chooses to describe it, cups should *never* hurt. The saying "no pain, no gain" is not the standard here, even if some types of bodywork may operate with this mindset. Cups can feel therapeutically intense (generally if stronger suction is used), but the best comparison to this type of intensity is to that of a trigger point or deep-tissue bodywork: on a scale of 1 to 10 (with 10 being the most painful), cups should never go past a 7 or 8 at their most intense. If cups hurt when applied, they can cause trauma, such as bruising.

suction in initial applications so the body has time to welcome any vacuum therapy, rather than overdoing it. Cupping is an entirely new concept of physical manipulation and the body needs time to respond to what has been changed, both in fluid exchanges and separation of previously adhered tissues. The more an individual uses cups, the more they can typically learn and anticipate the outcomes, but there can always be surprises or unexpected reactions. Reactions depend on a few variables — a person's level of hydration, activity, age, nutrition and previous experiences with bodywork — all of which can offer some insight as to how this individual will respond. For these reasons, I recommend limiting initial applications, as suggested below.

As a practitioner, I sometimes hear stories of people receiving cupping from a therapist for an hour during their first experience of this procedure. As a result of such excessive cupping, recipients may feel sick, tired and sore afterwards, or perhaps experience adverse tissue reactions, including bruising or swelling.

Consider these varying times when using cups the first time:

- If someone has never received a massage or bodywork, cups should be used gently and perhaps for only a few minutes.
- If someone is very dehydrated and their tissue is thick or very dense, cups should initially be applied gently to increase surface hydration before attempting any stronger suction. If there is no discomfort or change in the tissue, you may proceed to a deeper suction pressure, if desired. However, if the tissue feels thicker or denser after the cup is removed, do not work with any deeper suction at this time, as the movement of fluid has already been significant for this initial application.
- If someone receives regular bodywork, is well hydrated and exercises regularly, cups may be applied for longer periods and with perhaps stronger suction, but only if it is comfortable.

- If applying cups for a full body, lymphatic application, this treatment can last up to 1 hour. The suction pressure is light and the movements are gentle.

What should come after the first cupping procedure?

To assess the initial cupping visit, I suggest getting feedback from all recipients immediately after the procedure, as well as in the days that follow (this is even more highly suggested for more professional applications and environments where patient progress is being noted). Feedback allows the person applying the cups to know how their work was received and how to plan for the next application. Here are some examples of assessing an initial treatment:

- If someone felt better and experienced improvement or perhaps felt no major differences after their first treatment of cups, a longer treatment time or increased suction might be considered.
- If someone felt some fatigue, headache or nausea after their first treatment, there may have been too much toxic movement within their system. The next application should not increase in intensity and less cupping (pressure, time or both) is recommended.
- If someone felt a lot of pain, bruising or swelling after their treatment, the person applying the cups should not only lessen their next application, but also further evaluate the recipient for such measures as hydration, any overlooked contraindications, tissue integrity (such as vascular issues or weak muscle tone), overall health, etc.

There is no one expected outcome, so it is always best to approach each individual according to their own personal conditions.

How often can cups be used?

Cupping should not be done every day. Considering how disruptive cups can be to the pre-existing state of various body systems as well as to the amount of fluid exchange, it is important to allow the body time to process what has been affected before applying cups again. Some of the systems that could experience change include:

- **Lymphatic:** Cups are lifting and separating whatever structures may have been "stuck," which may have caused fluid retention or immobility in the first place. While cups are extremely helpful, using them too often can move too much fluid, ultimately causing swelling. The body should be allowed to process and settle for approximately 48 hours before reapplying cups to the same location.

- **Muscular:** While cups can yield good results in relieving pain and increasing the range of motion, the area cupped may be sensitive to what has been released. This is no different than deep-tissue therapies. How sensitive is the area the next day? Should it be worked again while in a state of discomfort? In these cases, the answer is no. Cups can be applied to different muscles in different locations, but it is strongly advised not to repeat an application in the same location within 48 hours.

How long will it take until something is "fixed" with cupping?

If this were an answerable question, cupping would be *the* miracle therapy! While cups can yield some truly extraordinary results, each person is different. Furthermore, because of cupping's non-invasive application and the systems involved in releasing restricted tissue, it may be best to approach the how long question in a more cumulative manner. This means that whatever condition you are working on (pain relief, spider veins, cellulite, scar tissue, etc.), a few weeks of regular applications is suggested. The condition can then be reassessed and a further treatment plan created from there, if necessary. Chances are that if something has accumulated over a few years (for example, cellulite), it will take at least a few weeks of constant applications to have major changes happen. However, one treatment can yield excellent (and sometimes shocking!) results.

Where is the evidence that cupping actually works like you say it does?

As with any non-invasive therapy (massage therapy, physical therapy, acupuncture), the proof is often in the results. Western medicinal practices depend on (or at least want) proof, while Eastern practices look for results. Cupping is a complementary and alternative medicine (CAM) therapy, which has its own mysticism as well as its skeptics. The search for factual proof of cupping's efficacy is similar to that for many alternative therapies and can be limited in clinical documentation and often inconclusive. The fact that cups have been employed the world over for thousands of years, however, speaks volumes for its efficacy, as do the thousands of cases and testimonials accrued by this therapy. The Russian Ministry of Health has done more than 40 years of research and established its official use in its medical system. The "proof" is in the work and its results.

Safety Point

Do not reapply cups until any marking has disappeared. Cupping marks may last a few hours to a few days — the more intense the release, the longer the mark may remain and should be left to process. Lymphatic drainage treatments should not be marking the skin, so those can be done approximately every 48 hours.

The Efficacy of Cupping Through Thermographics

Thermographic imaging uses different colors to display the levels of activity in an area. The cooler the colors, the less circulation or activity is present in various body tissues in that region. The blue tones indicate cold or lack of circulation, while other colors indicate the progression of temperatures from cold to hot — dark green to green, yellow, orange and red, with white as the color of most heat (compare the expression "white hot") or the degree of inflammation.

In this series of images, we follow a subject who was experiencing upper right shoulder pain, which was also contributing to her neck pain. She also complained of an overall feeling of not being well, as she had just returned from a trip to a very cold place.

Following the cupping treatment, here is reaction from the subject, who had never experienced cupping before these images were taken:

"I felt so much better following the procedure. Although I felt a little sore, the soreness turned to relief, my muscles being much more relaxed and my neck in much less pain. I slept better than I had in days, woke up and felt so warm! I felt the warmth most of the day, and still a lot less sore than I had been before the treatment."

PICTURE 1, BEFORE TREATMENT. TIME STAMPED IMAGE, 2:08 P.M.

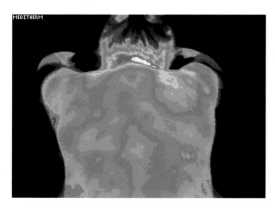

Note her top right shoulder region with the localized heat and the white-hot tension in her neck. Also, her mid-thoracic spine shows signs of irritation (lighter green along the spine and to the right of it), indicating tension within the lower shoulder muscles and around the spine, compensating for the pain she was feeling in the areas above. Also note the imbalance of circulation.

PICTURE 2, FOLLOWING THE FIRST APPLICATION OF CUPS. TIME STAMPED IMAGE, 2:11 P.M.

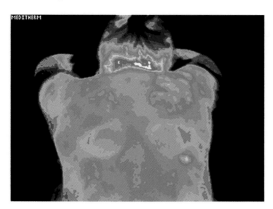

Six stationary cups were applied (three along each side of the spine) from the base of the neck to the mid-thoracic spine. While most of the region remains unchanged, the general surface has become cooler. Notice the two blue circle-like shapes in her mid-back region, where the largest two cups were placed?

PICTURE 3, AFTER 10 MINUTES OF MOVING CUPS WITH SLOW, METHODICAL MOVEMENTS AND LIGHT–TO–MEDIUM–SUCTION PRESSURE ALL OVER HER UPPER BODY. TIME STAMPED IMAGE, 2:21 P.M.

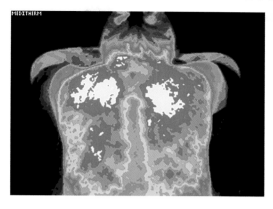

Note the major increase in surface heat levels due to the increased blood flow drawn into the area. Also note how it drew the excessive heat/inflammation *down* and out of the neck.

PICTURE 4, NO CUPS USED (SHE WAS RESTING). TIME STAMPED IMAGE, 2:24 P.M.

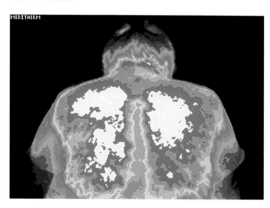

Circulation increased on its own when the body was left to process the cupping for a few minutes; the increased vasodilation *naturally* allowed for circulation to expand into the area.

PICTURE 5, NO CUPPING DONE, CIRCULATION RECEDING AFTER THE TREATMENT. TIME STAMPED IMAGE, 2:30 P.M.

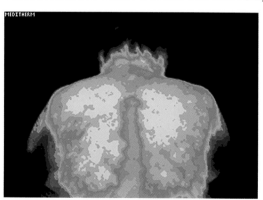

Note an even distribution of overall circulation, as well as a decrease of tension in the original areas of complaint and a decrease of tension along the mid-thoracic spine.

CHAPTER 3

Therapeutic Benefits on the Body Systems

THE HUMAN BODY

Human anatomy is extremely complex and functions in an incredibly harmonious manner. The intricate nature of the various body systems has been the subject of countless books and endless research, as well as the focus of many dedicated fields of health care.

While it may seem like only one body system at a time is being targeted when cups are applied, multiple systems are also affected whenever this technique is used. This chapter will simplify how every layer of tissue, blood vessel and organ is interconnected, and why there is no "one cup application" for any condition, nor identical applications for any two different people. Regulating internal body temperatures, for example, involves several body systems (muscular, circulatory, integumentary), and cupping can directly benefit all of them simultaneously in a very logical and cohesive manner. In fact, because cupping can penetrate up to 4 inches (10 cm) deep into the body, every system can be affected to some degree by cup applications. Some systems may be more affected than others (circulatory system versus reproductive system); however, it is important to know the potential benefits that cupping can offer throughout the entire body.

TISSUES OF THE BODY

The four major types of tissue in the human body are:

- Epithelial
- Connective
- Muscular
- Nervous

Epithelial and connective tissues cross several body systems. Unless specified as muscle tissue, the two types of body tissues referenced in this book are the following:

Epithelial Tissue

- Covers our entire body (skin)
- Lines certain visceral organs, blood vessels and body cavities; any organ that has direct exposure to the outside elements, such as the oral cavity and esophagus

- Surrounds glands of the body (such as endocrine and exocrine)

Functions: Epithelial tissue, such as the skin, protects the internal environment of our body; absorbs various substances, such as vitamin D from the sun and nutrients in the small intestines; filters materials before entering the body, such as dirt and particles out of the air we breathe in the respiratory tract; secretes various substances, such as enzymes, hormones and bodily fluids; excretes fluids, such as perspiration from the sweat glands; and diffuses different fluids, such as blood during capillary exchange.

Epithelial tissue is avascular (lacking blood vessels) and receives blood from connecting blood vessels by diffusion. It has one surface exposed and the other attached to connective tissue.

Connective Tissue

- Most tissues in the body are connective tissue
- Exists in a matrix design, which allows for a lot of space within its cellular structure

Functions: Connective tissue supports and protects body structure; distributes nutrients; supports immune defense; and prevents blood loss (clotting). Most connective tissue has a strong blood supply (vascular). With its matrix design, this space allows for all kinds of interstitial debris (for example, old blood) to pass through and risk becoming embedded.

Connective tissue is responsible for the formation of blood, the dermis (inner layer of skin), superficial and deep fascia (fibrous tissue that keeps everything attached and connected), adipose tissue (stores energy and provides cushioning), bones, cartilage, ligaments, tendons and other thick, connective tissue structures such as aponeuroses, tendons and periosteum (see next page).

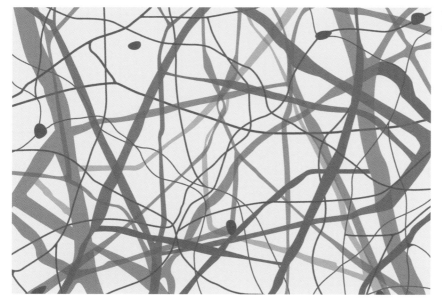

Cellular matrix of connective tissue

Connective Tissue Structures to Know

Ligaments connect bones.

Tendons connect muscle to bone.

Periosteum is connective tissue that encompasses bones (except the ends, where cartilage is found).

Cartilage lines the ends of bones where they meet in a joint.

Fascia is a connective tissue that literally connects everything in the body. This tissue:

- Sections off muscles.
- Keeps visceral organs in place.
- Maintains structural integrity.

   Without it, we would not have the body form we do, but rather a pile of goo on the ground!

Aponeurosis is a strong, thin sheet of connective tissue that has functions similar to tendons or fascia.

- Like a tendon, it connects muscle to muscle or muscle to bone.
- Like fascia, it keeps muscles bundled or organs contained together within a certain region.

   While the human body contains many aponeuroses, some of the primary ones are located:

- Over the crown of the head
- Along the spine
- In the abdominal region
- In the palm
- In the sole of the foot

   For more information on **muscle** and **nerve** tissues, see pages 47 and 63, respectively.

BODY SYSTEMS

Therapeutic cupping can be directed to address one body system, such as the muscular system, more than another, but remember, the entire body is one interconnected unit, one system. This section will isolate each system of the body, define its functions and note any potential issues and how cupping can affect or help improve them.

INTEGUMENTARY SYSTEM

ANATOMY

The integumentary system is composed of skin, hair, nails and glands (oil and sweat).

The skin is a permeable barrier, capable of both excreting and absorbing substances. The skin can help regulate body temperature and promote detoxification through perspiration. However, this same exposure mechanism leaves our bodies open and vulnerable to invasive external pathogens, such as carbon dioxide, noxious fumes, organic solvent and chemicals, and countless other skin irritants (for example, poison ivy). Consider the vulnerability to any invasive substance: cold, wind, negative energies.

The skin is also an extension of the nervous system, as it is the first line of communication to the outside world. Reactions to pressure, pain, temperature and environmental elements are first introduced to the body here. From this initial contact, information travels along the peripheral nerves to the central nervous system for proper evaluation and subsequent reaction.

FUNCTIONS

- To protect the internal environment of the body from all external substances.
- To excrete and absorb substances; skin is a two-way barrier.
- To communicate initial sensory input to the central nervous system.

What's Under the Skin?

The *epidermis* is the outermost layer, housing pores and hair follicles, and contains no blood vessels.

The *dermis* is just below the epidermis and is made up of connective tissue. This layer contains sensory receptors (nerve endings; see Anatomy FYI, page 37), some adipose tissue and the blood vessels that supply blood to and remove waste from the epidermis.

The *hypodermis* is the deepest layer of the skin and is made up of superficial fascia and adipose tissue. While the hypodermis is not considered a true "layer" of skin, it provides the connection between the integumentary system and the underlying muscular system.

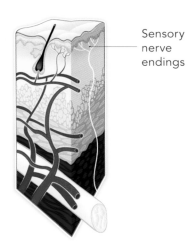

Sensory
nerve
endings

Skin is thicker on the back of the body than the front, is at its thickest on the hands and feet, and is thinnest around the eyes. The skin is the largest organ in the body, yet it is the last one to receive blood. The only way to supply blood to the epidermis comes from capillaries connected directly to the underlying dermis, through a process called capillary exchange (supplies blood while removing waste; see "Circulatory System," page 38, for more information).

Body Temperature Regulation

The sudoriferous glands, or sweat glands, are also located in the dermis and help remove excessive heat from the body. When internal temperatures rise, overall circulation increases and urges these glands to produce and release sweat to help cool the body down.

Nerve Endings

The dermis houses various mechanoreceptors, which are nerve endings of the peripheral nervous system (see Anatomy FYI, opposite). Whenever something touches the body, these receptors transmit this initial sense of contact along the peripheral nerves to the brain, where the brain processes this information and forms a response accordingly.

Here's how they work: Too much pressure from a massage can elicit one response (such as a verbal request to lighten up or a "wincing" response within the muscles to tighten up and protect the body), while soft, soothing touch can bring about another (stimulating the parasympathetic nervous system and promoting relaxation). See page 62 for more information on the nervous system.

CONSTANT NERVE ENDING IRRITATION

Sometimes, surface tissues can be locked in a state of constant irritation for a variety of reasons. Two opposite extremes are cellulite (a concentration of adipose cells and connective tissue restrictions

DID YOU KNOW?

The body works best when internal temperatures stay within a relative range. When temperatures change, the body works to regulate this through combined efforts of the integumentary, circulatory and muscular systems.

that can create irregular tension on these nerve endings, causing an altered response to touch) or more serious conditions like fibromyalgia (some cases have increased numbers of nerve endings around capillaries that may be easily irritated; see Chapter 5: "Safe Cupping" for more insight about fibromyalgia). Any constant irritation of these nerve endings can contribute to chronic pain patterns.

Whether the surface tensions are altered by systemic irritations (fibromyalgia) or from tissue damage (such as burns), the dermis is most comfortable when it is loose, pliable and hydrated. Anything else can cause distress and discomfort.

Safety Point

These same irritated nerve endings will quickly respond to too much suction pressure; therefore, refrain from applying stronger suction initially. Rather, just as with massage therapy, work slowly into any strong pressure.

Anatomy FYI

Nerve endings of the peripheral nervous system are known as *sensory receptors*; they collect input and send it to the brain to elicit a proper response. Nociceptors are located throughout the body, especially near the surface. These nerve endings respond to pain. Mechanoreceptors are located within the dermis and detect different sensations, such as pain, vibration and various applied pressures. Thermoreceptors are located just under the surface of the skin. They respond to temperatures (hot and cold).

How Cupping Affects the Integumentary System

- **Stimulates superficial circulation.** The suction pump effect of cups stimulates the general distribution and recirculation of blood and superficial lymph fluids. Enhancing this microcirculation improves overall surface tissue health and appearance.
- **Supports temperature regulation.** Because of the enhanced vasodilation and the drawing of fluids to the surface, cups help support the excreting actions that occur within the skin (for example, sweat), which in turn optimize systemic function. This doesn't mean that cupping will make you sweat. Rather, it promotes optimal functioning of such processes.
- **Desensitizes superficial pain patterns.** Relief can be brought to these potentially aggravated nerve endings by applying simple, gentle cupping. Like the relaxing and soothing sensations simple massage strokes of the hand offer these nerve endings, gently *lifting* rather than pressing on the tissue can provoke some equally comforting responses.

ANATOMY

The circulatory system is composed of the heart, blood and blood vessels, lymph and lymph vessels and lymph glands (tonsils, spleen, thymus).

The circulatory system is a crucial part of health and well-being. Its primary function is to keep fluids moving throughout the body.

There are two divisions of the circulatory system: cardiovascular and lymphvascular.

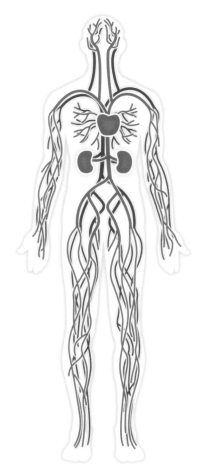

The Cardiovascular System

FUNCTIONS

- Supports a systemic distribution of respiratory gases (oxygen and carbon dioxide), nutrients, antibodies and hormones (from the endocrine system).
- Supports immune system functions by producing disease-fighting cells such as white blood cells and aiding in the removal of any unhealthy substances or waste materials, such as viruses.

- Protects the body from excessive loss of bodily fluids from trauma with the mechanism of blood clotting.
- Helps regulate body temperature by moving heat from active muscles to skin via dilated blood vessels, where it can be dissipated through sweat.

Blood Circulation

The cardiovascular system contains the heart, blood and blood vessels. The heart acts as a central pump to move blood through the vessels to every cell of the body. The arteries carry nutrient-rich, oxygenated blood away from the heart for anatomical distribution. As arteries start to branch out, they become thinner in composition (called arterioles) and eventually reach the most distal points and become very thin in structure (called capillaries). The primary function of capillaries is capillary exchange.

Anatomy FYI

Proximal is a term used to describe any point that is *closer to* the torso, or another designated location on the body. *Distal* is a term used to describe any point that is *further away from* the torso, or another designated location on the body.

The carotid artery in the neck is more *proximal* to the heart than the femoral artery, located in the thigh. Capillaries are the most *distal* segments of arteries.

Capillary Exchange

Capillaries are the most distal end of an artery. They exist in almost every tissue of the body. Their membrane walls are very thin and permeable, which allows for diffusion to take place.

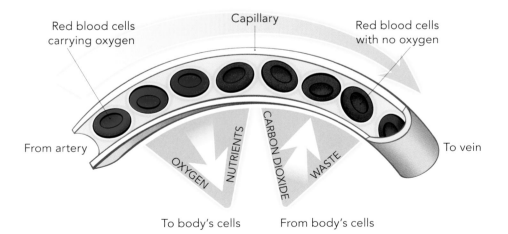

Capillary exchange is the process of diffusion in which blood and nutrients are distributed to the surrounding tissue while waste from cells and interstitial fluids are removed simultaneously. These are crucial components of a healthy circulatory system's function. Capillary networks are highly concentrated in muscles and organs, and are more sporadic within connective tissues.

Venous Return

Veins remove blood low in oxygen from these distal points (the smallest parts of veins are called venules) where capillaries end and return it to the heart by a process called venous return. Veins do not have the full-strength assistance of the heart for moving fluid like arteries do, and therefore work harder for the return process. Instead, veins have flap valves, which open only in the direction of the heart and stop backflow if necessary. Veins also rely on muscle contractions in the limbs to encourage this venous return. Blood is ultimately recirculated back to the heart through the combination of the flap valve system, muscular contractions and pressure changes within the torso from organ functions (such as lungs from respiration).

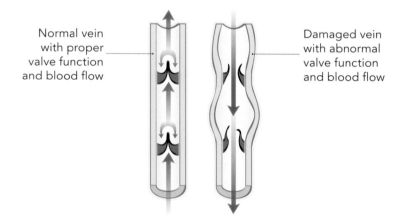

Normal vein with proper valve function and blood flow

Damaged vein with abnormal valve function and blood flow

Venous return is a bit more challenging than blood distribution. Veins not only have to work against gravity for recirculation, but their flap valve system also requires support because of the overall delicate nature of their flap valves. If too much stress is put solely on the function of the flap valves and they don't have enough support — for example, when there is insufficient muscle activity in the limbs — it can overload the system and challenge the natural opening and closing functions of the valves, potentially rendering them damaged or incapacitated. This poor recirculation process can cause damage to the veins. Veins are closer to the surface than arteries, however, so their function can be more easily influenced and supported by outside efforts. Considering the crucial role of muscle contractions in venous return, exercise and manual therapies like massage are key in optimal overall circulation.

Body Temperature Regulation

The cardiovascular system also functions to regulate the body's temperature. The body will dilate its vessels (vasodilation) to allow for heat to escape, or it will constrict the same vessels when the internal temperature is too low to contain heat inside the body. If too cold, the body will initiate a vibration within the muscles to stimulate more heat, a response known as shivering.

The body works best when internal temperatures stay within a relative range. When temperatures change, the body works to regulate this through combined efforts of the integumentary, circulatory and muscular systems.

Safety Point

Cupping should not be applied strongly over *any* superficial vascular bodies (arteries, veins), so their vital functions are not interrupted.

How Cupping Affects the Cardiovascular System

- **Promotes overall circulation.** Capillaries are the slowest blood-moving segments in the cardiovascular system, and the ability to influence their exchange processes with cupping is very valuable. Cupping promotes dilation of these tiny vessels and encourages distribution of fluids through to their end points. The increased distribution of blood, oxygen and nutrients at such a microscopic level is crucial for optimal overall health. Increased microcirculation improves general circulation — the greater the output of blood, the stronger the return becomes.
- **Encourages venous return.** Think of how cups lift the tissue and how veins are more superficial than arteries. Gentle cupping can help flap valves perform their functions, while working the cups in a centripetal direction (toward the trunk of the body) can offer significant support in venous return.
- **Affects blood pressure.** The vasodilation and systemic circulation that cupping enhances can lead to a decrease in vascular pressure. This can be beneficial for both high and low blood pressure, but be sure that suction pressure isn't too aggressive in either case. Those with low blood pressure may feel a little dizzy after cupping due to the sudden "rush" in their circulation.
- **Influences body temperature.** With cupping's effect on vasodilation, temperatures can be altered quite easily. While this is beneficial in helping to regulate internal body temperatures when it's too hot, it can also expose the internal environment to accepting cold temperatures from outside (remember, the skin is a two-way permeable barrier). Monitor body temperatures for a short time after cupping therapies.

The Lymphvascular System

ANATOMY

The lymphvascular, or lymphatic, system contains the lymph, lymph vessels and lymph glands and organs (tonsils, adenoids, spleen and thymus).

FUNCTIONS

One of the primary functions of the lymphatic system is to maintain balance in the volume of bodily fluids. Any displaced fluids (from blood distribution, see "What Is Lymph?," next page) go back into the blood to maintain regular blood volume and pressure. Without this return, both blood volume and pressure will decrease substantially. If this fluid remains, the interstitial spaces expand, thereby creating edema, or swelling. If the lymphatic system becomes overloaded, then swelling can remain and the entire lymphatic system goes out of balance while trying to remedy this excessive fluid stagnation. The lymphatic system's work is constant and absolutely vital to maintaining the balance of bodily fluids. Keeping lymph fluid circulating helps support overall health.

ADDITIONAL FUNCTIONS

- Filters lymph fluids and pathogenic substances, offering major defensive support to the immune system.
- Transports fats and some vitamins from the digestive system to blood circulation.

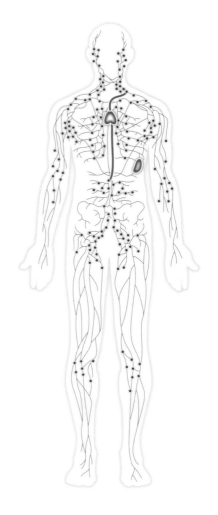

What Is Lymph?

The circulation of blood within the cardiovascular system addresses 90 percent of the body's fluid exchange processes. However, the 10 percent of fluid that escapes venous return remains in the space between tissues (interstitial or extracellular fluids), and this is where lymph is formed. In other words, lymph is any material that cannot be reabsorbed into veins due to its different composition, whether it is certain protein molecules, cellular waste or foreign substances, such as bacteria.

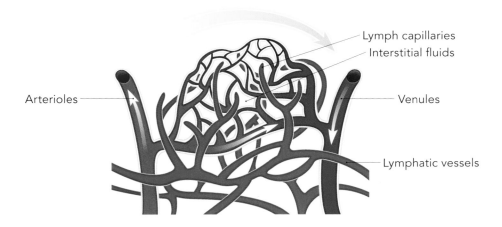

Arterioles — Lymph capillaries — Interstitial fluids — Venules — Lymphatic vessels

Lymph Capillaries

The most superficial structures of this system, called lymph capillaries, lie just under the surface of the skin. These capillaries *start* at the most distal points near the skin, similar to how capillaries of the cardiovascular system reach these most distal points. Lymph capillaries, however, work in one direction, have no central pump (like the heart) to move fluids and rely solely on outside influences to create this movement. Visceral organ movements, skeletal muscle contractions and respiratory functions offer similar support to the lymphvascular system as they do to the venous return of the cardiovascular system.

The lymph capillaries have their own unique type of flap valve-like structures. These flaps respond to external pressure and open to allow lymph to enter the system. When an excess of interstitial fluid is creating this pressure on the flap valves, they open and try to accommodate as much of this waste material as possible. If the volume of this fluid exceeds maximum capacity, however, the system cannot take it all in, causing a sort of systemic backup or stagnation, for example in the case of edema or swelling.

DID YOU KNOW?

Fluids that exist in the superficial lymph capillaries have no designated direction and can be easily influenced. Manual therapy, such as massage or manual lymph drainage, is very effective in encouraging lymphatic drainage.

Lymph Movement

Lymph moves in one direction, toward the subclavian veins in the upper chest, where it rejoins circulation. As the lymphatic system progresses deeper into the body and further toward its core, the structures become larger and more complex: from superficial lymph capillaries, they grow into lymph vessels. These lymph vessels have flap valves more similar to those within veins that prevent any backflow. Lymph vessels develop into lymph nodes where much of the lymph is filtered. What remains is fed into lymph trunks, and eventually into the two main drainage ducts in the torso (right thoracic duct and [left] thoracic duct).

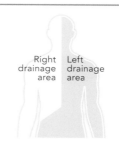

Anatomy FYI

Located under the clavicle (collarbones), the *right thoracic duct* drains lymph from the right arm, right side of the head and right half of the torso into the right subclavian vein. The *(left) thoracic duct* drains lymph from the rest of the body into the left subclavian vein.

Right drainage area   Left drainage area

The entire body has a directional "map" of how lymph flows into the thoracic ducts. We have superficial drainage pathways and slightly deeper, or intermediate, drainage pathways that have similar routes, but they vary somewhat and should be addressed accordingly, depending on certain physical conditions (for example, oncology patients). See Chapter 9: "Therapeutic Cupping for Lymphatic Drainage" for more information on drainage pathways and how to work more specifically with this system.

Immune System

The lymphatic system is also the first line of defense against illness-causing pathogens, such as bacteria, viruses, parasites and so on. Any pathogenic substance that enters the body can be discovered in the same interstitial space where the lymph fluid originates. While white blood cells (leukocytes) are formed in the bone marrow, they change into defensive cells called lymphocytes once they enter the lymphatic system. As white blood cells specific to the lymphatic system, certain lymphocytes (like T cells, or thymus-produced cells) identify invasive materials and then strategize various attack procedures, such as initiating the release of certain bio-chemicals (like cytokines) to launch appropriate attack responses, or activating the production of antibodies (antibodies like B cells, or bone marrow cells), which identify these infectious cells found within the system, directing the T cells and other destructive lymphocytes where to attack. They proceed to attack these foreign substances, such as bacteria, as soon as they are detected, then lymph capillaries begin the process of removing the waste to the larger vessels (lymph nodes). With all this extraordinary cellular activity, swelling can occur wherever this is happening, such as swollen lymph nodes or sites of local infection. If an injury, such as a sprained ankle or knee surgery, is the cause of swelling, similar lymphatic "emergency response" cells are triggered and directed to do their job locally.

Safety Point

During times of acute infection — whether from bacteria or virus — cupping should not be used around these local sites of swelling. (See Chapter 9 for more information on when to use cups if the lymphatic system is challenged, as well as "Working with Inflammation" in Chapter 10.)

Types of White Blood Cells

There are five types of white blood cells:

- Neutrophils (most common)
- Eosinophils
- Basophils
- Monocytes
- Lymphocytes

B lymphocytes, or B cells, produce antibodies that mark invasive cells (virus, bacteria) for attack. T lymphocytes, or T cells, are then sent to destroy the antibody–identified invasive cells.

Nutrient Distribution

The abdomen contains a high volume of blood and lymph capillaries, especially around the digestive organs. Along with many blood capillaries, specialized lymph capillaries, called lacteals, surround the small intestines in particular. When foods are broken down here, nutrients are extracted and mostly taken into the bloodstream by the blood capillaries. The lacteals are designed to absorb essential fats and subsequently take them into the lymphatic system, where these fats are processed and eventually distributed into the bloodstream.

How Cupping Affects the Lymphvascular System

- **Encourages lymph drainage.** This is one of the greatest benefits of therapeutic cupping. Keep in mind that cups lift tissue rather than press it, so the flap valves contained within this delicate system respond positively to this therapy. Whether assisting in the removal of lymph from within layers of soft tissue, such as removing waste from within tight muscles, or moving lymph along its drainage route, cups are very beneficial to overall lymphatic health.
- **Affects overall lymphatic movement.** Working the surface very lightly will have a direct effect on the deeper structures contained within the lymphatic system. The system responds in a suction pump-like response to even the lightest superficial stimulation, which means that just stimulating the surface (without strong pressure) will have a direct effect on everything underneath it.
- **Encourages directional movement.** Because of the superficial lymphatic system's lack of direction, the lightest therapeutic cupping can encourage the direction of flow. This explains why it is so important to work in a centripetal direction on the limbs with cups. Think of a cup full of water — wherever you move it, the fluid will follow.
- **Supports deeper lymphatic drainage.** Addressing the slightly deeper, or intermediate, lymph vessels, gentle therapeutic cupping can encourage their flap valves to open and move fluids along, just as they do with the blood in the veins. Cups can also gather up excessive lymph (remember, it has no heart pumping it to make movement) and remove it from the interstitial spaces where it may lie stagnant.
- **Supports immune system functions.** At a cellular level, overall immune system functions begin within the lymphatic system. White blood cells work to destroy and absorb pathogenic substances and foreign debris, and cupping can support the regional removal of the waste material offered by lymphatic drainage so the lymphocytes can continue to do their job. Cups should *not,* however, be worked over the area of immune-fighting activity. Rather, when the time is right, cups should be applied above the area, encouraging movement in the direction of where lymph is going.
- **Addresses general abdominal congestion.** Gentle cupping in the abdomen can help clear lymphatic stagnation, and this can help with overall health.

How Cupping Affects the Total Circulatory System

Cupping initiates a simultaneous reaction of lymph fluid and blood: both fluids are drawn into the area where the cup is applied. This is an important concept to understand. While a stationary cup may be applied to feed blood to an ischemic area (an area with a lack of blood flow), you don't want to draw too much lymph into the area. Applications that are too long or strong may *create* stagnation; that is, "clog" an area rather than encourage the movement of fluids within the layers being treated.

MUSCULAR SYSTEM

ANATOMY

The muscular system is composed entirely of soft tissue: muscles (skeletal, smooth and cardiac), tendons and fascia.

FUNCTIONS

- Moves the body.
- Maintains posture and stability.
- Supports overall circulation, including lymph movement.
- Controls smooth muscle movements of visceral organs.
- Supports body temperature regulation.

Muscle Tissues

There are three different types of muscle tissue: skeletal, smooth and cardiac.

Skeletal muscle tissue makes up the muscles that control the movement and stability of the human body.
- Controls voluntary muscle contractions
- Muscle fibers are striated
- Attaches to bones, connective tissue and other muscles

Smooth muscle tissue is found in the visceral organs.
- Controls involuntary muscle contractions
- Muscle fibers are long, designed for slow, sustained contractions and require little energy to perform their work
- Surrounds visceral organs

Cardiac muscle tissue is found only in the heart.
- Controls involuntary muscle contractions
- Muscle fibers are striated
- Makes up the walls of the heart

Cupping can affect skeletal and smooth muscles, so this section will address these two types.

Anatomy FYI

Involuntary muscles are controlled by the autonomic nervous system without conscious effort. These muscles control the work of all the visceral organs. *Voluntary muscles* are controlled by a conscious effort, meaning you have to initiate their actions with intention. These muscles are known as your skeletal muscles, the muscles that move your body.

Skeletal Muscle Tissue

The human body contains more than 600 muscles, which vary in length and size and surround most of the skeletal structure.

Skeletal muscle tissues are organized in parallel rows and are created by complex layering of various muscle fibers and connective tissues, with blood and lymph vessels woven in between. Epimysium is the thickest connective tissue in muscle formation, enveloping the entire muscle and separating one muscle grouping from another (for example, separating the biceps femoris from the sartorius muscle in the quadriceps of the thigh). The epimysium also continues past the end of these designated muscles to become the tendons associated with the muscles.

TYPES OF CONNECTIVE TISSUE

There are three major types of connective tissue involved in muscle tissue formation:

- The innermost muscle fibers are bundled together by a thin layer of connective tissue called *endomysium*.
- These small bundles (called *fascicles*) are then grouped together and surrounded by another layer of connective tissue called *perimysium*.
- All these bundled fibers are finally grouped together and enveloped by yet another layer of connective tissue called *epimysium*.

Anatomy FYI

Mechanoreceptors are nerve endings of the peripheral nervous system. *Proprioceptors* are specialized mechanoreceptors associated only with muscles, tendons and joint. They respond to changes in muscle length, tension, position, pain and blood pressure.

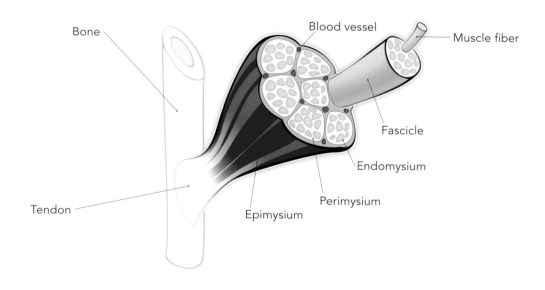

Tendons

Tendons are condensed cords of connective tissue with minimal blood supply that attach skeletal muscles to bones, fascia or other connective tissue structures, such as the iliotibial (IT) band.

Fascia

The muscular system's anatomy is medically defined as being composed of three types of muscle tissue and tendons — all being forms of connective tissue — yet there is no specific mention of fascia, a complex and vital component of the human anatomy.

Fascia is a form of connective tissue involved whenever the body is manipulated. There is no specific reason as to how fascia weaves its way through the body. From the surface of the skin to the density of bones and everything in between, its structure is organized chaos. Fascia works to hold the entire body together for overall balanced health and well-being, known as homeostasis.

Master myofascial physical therapist John F. Barnes says, "There is no such thing as a muscle," and if you think about a muscle's composition, this claim has considerable merit. Every muscle is formed, surrounded and compartmentalized by fascia. While muscle tissues make up the anatomy, fascia creates the structure and stability of any muscle formation, and fascial restrictions are easily discovered within the muscular system. Fascia is highly permeable, and fluid is constantly passing through it. Whenever a "kink" appears in the human body (for example, in the case of repetitive motion injuries or as the result of sleeping patterns or impact injuries), fascia reorganizes to help maintain balance and order, and adhesions can often occur. If fascial adhesions go unaddressed, local dysfunction may lead to a surrounding disorder and can potentially lead to an array of physical ailments.

> **DID YOU KNOW?**
>
> Fascia is a complicated structure and has been extensively researched. While this chapter highlights only the pertinent points related to cupping, much is available from training programs by John F. Barnes, PT (www.myofascialrelease.com) and Anatomy Trains (www.anatomytrains.com), as well as Dr. Jean-Claude Guimberteau's research and book (with Colin Armstrong), *Architecture of Human Living Fascia*.

How Skeletal Muscles Work

Skeletal muscles work to move the body as well as create stability. Skeletal muscle responses are voluntary and therefore activated by the brain.

These muscles have a rich supply of nerves, blood and lymph capillaries and require continual circulation of blood as well as lymph removal for optimal performance. For these reasons, they rely on a large amount of oxygen, which they use to access stored ATP (adenosine triphosphate) to engage movements.

If skeletal muscles are too tight or restricted, or waste is not properly being removed, then these fundamental functions can be severely diminished.

Muscle Energy Production

Energy is normally produced when ATP, an energy-producing substance that is stored in the muscle cells, is broken down and released into the system. The two methods of accessing this energy, called aerobic and anaerobic metabolism, produce their own waste materials. (For more information on energy production for muscular activity, see "Athletic Performance and Cupping," page 230.)

Aerobic metabolism uses oxygen to release ATP. The body uses oxygen along with glucose to access this stored ATP energy. Once finished, the waste products are carbon dioxide, which is removed from the body by exhalation, and water, released as sweat when the body is overheated.

Anaerobic respiration uses only glucose rather than oxygen to release ATP. Without oxygen, the body breaks down glucose to produce pyruvate, which accesses this stored ATP. Once finished, the waste products are lactic acid and heat.

The body has a naturally high reproduction rate of ATP, which leads to a sort of never-ending supply of energy.

Both processes occur in the body whenever energy is required by muscle tissue. During basic daily activities or short-term cardiovascular exercise, aerobic metabolism is active and uses oxygen (as well as some glucose) to create energy production. During vigorous exercise, anaerobic metabolism is active and the body begins using glucose to start the chain of energy-producing events. Whether aerobic or anaerobic, energy production creates waste, such as heat and lactic acid, as well as other metabolic wastes, such as protons, which are the "garbage" left by the broken-down ATP. The muscles naturally try to expel all this waste via lymph drainage, but this may be hindered when muscles become tight.

PROBLEMS WITH TRAPPED WASTE

- If metabolic waste, such as lactic acid or protons, is not purged, it remains stagnant in muscles. If this stagnation remains, it can

Glycolysis is a complex chemical process of breaking down glucose in the bloodstream — from the food you eat — to produce energy. *Pyruvate* is a product of this process and is used to access ATP for energy production. During anaerobic metabolism, pyruvate converts into lactate, which remains in the muscles to enable the energy-production process to continue without oxygen.

block the replenishment of oxygen and alter the chemical balance in muscle tissue and lead to a more acidic environment, called acidosis. These combined elements can create added pressure on the nerve endings in the muscle, triggering a pain response known as the "burn" often used to describe overexerted muscles. All this can contribute to slow recovery times and hindered performances.

- If heat is not removed from the body, it remains trapped in the layers of muscle, leading to dehydration, and inevitably muscle tissues get "stuck," creating adhesions. These adhesions hinder optimal waste removal and rehydration from returning to the spaces between normal layers of muscle tissue, which can lead to chronic edema if the displaced fluids are not properly addressed. Over time, these adhesions can lead to bigger restrictions, which in turn can limit full range of motion and functioning.

Building Muscle

To build stronger muscles, necessary microtraumas occur within the muscle tissue. Every time muscles are strength-trained, they are torn. The body responds with the same type of inflammatory "emergency response" as it does to any trauma (see "Working with Inflammation" in Chapter 10 for more information), but the level of intensity varies. The more serious the strain injury, the greater the response effort. The smaller, necessary tears in muscle tissue stimulate minimum inflammation responses that initiate the rebuilding process of the smallest muscle fibers, called myofibrils.

Once activated, these reinforced myofibrils replicate, becoming thicker and stronger, rebuild muscle tissue at the site of the damage and increase the size of overall muscle tissue. However, this newly constructed, enriched muscle tissue is a form of scar tissue, considering its deviation from the natural muscle fibers. It is important to manipulate these irregular muscles as they grow so they only grow *with* the length of muscle, rather than stray from the natural grain of muscle fibers as scar tissue tends to do.

Anatomy FYI

Muscle strains are injuries suffered by muscle tissue or tendons. They're categorized as

- *1st degree:* Minimal tissue damage. Mild, localized pain and most of normal function is maintained. The tearing that occurs during muscle tissue reconstruction should be *below* a 1st degree strain.
- *2nd degree:* More serious tissue damage, possibly visible and palpable (marked by sensitivity to touch). More intense pain with some swelling and limited function.
- *3rd degree:* Total separation of tissue, clear visible damage to area. Severe pain with swelling, majority of function inhibited.

Creating Waste

The process of building muscle tissue has its own waste, which needs to be purged from the area like any other waste material. The waste in this instance, however, is the torn pieces of muscle tissue that were displaced at the time of injury. While the muscle tries to expel this waste via the lymph system like every other waste product, the tightness of newer, stronger muscles can inhibit this removal process in the same way tight muscles can interrupt the removal of waste from aerobic and anaerobic metabolism. This can also create a backup in lymphatic drainage, contributing to a stagnation of old blood tissue in the muscles. As muscles engage, they naturally pump blood through the area while simultaneously wringing out lymph, which removes metabolic waste, such as lactic acid, that is produced by such activities. Having well-hydrated, pliable muscle tissue allows these actions to perform at their best.

Tightness

Feeling tightness or stiffness is a general description of discomforts associated with skeletal muscles and is often caused by lack of optimal circulation and flexibility, for whatever reason. Any tightness or restriction of skeletal muscles can reduce function or overall performance if, for example, a nerve becomes compressed or tissue becomes ischemic (lacking blood flow). If tissue goes without necessary blood circulation, necrosis will occur. Prolonged lack of usage can eventually lead to a wasting away of skeletal muscle tissue, called atrophy.

Trigger Points

Commonly known as knots, trigger points are a concentrated area of soft tissue tightness and pain. Trigger points are problematic, whether caused by injury, internal responses to stress, postural imbalances or other causes, and can contribute to a great deal of physical discomfort. If a trigger point is in a skeletal muscle, the fibers are very tight and ischemic and can lead to pressure on the nerves, thereby triggering a pain response from the brain. Manual therapies often hold sustained pressure over these areas to promote local vasodilation, thereby stimulating blood flow, and the direct pressure encourages the muscle tissue to lengthen and relax.

Injured Tissue

When tissue damage occurs, skeletal muscles have the capability of relative regeneration (depending on the severity of injury), rushing blood and necessary inflammatory substances to the injured area. The body, however, must also maintain its inherent muscular functions (such as maintaining postural balance or daily activities) that are controlled by the brain.

DID YOU KNOW?

Trigger points can often have a phantom–like referral pattern. When touched, the person can have pain in a completely different area of the body — a phenomenon that illustrates how intertwined are our bodies: muscles, fascia, nerves, energy.

Anatomy FYI

Strains are damaged skeletal muscle tissues or tendons. *Sprains* are damaged ligaments.

When tissue damage is present, the entire soft tissue system is forced to prioritize its functions. While it makes an effort to rush healthy blood to the damaged tissue, it has to be sure to engage the skeletal muscle actions dictated by the brain. This creates the need to appropriate alternative routes of blood flow around the damage site, in turn causing the tissues immediately adjacent to become deficient in their blood flow. In this process, a vicious cycle is created: both the injured muscles and those directly adjacent to them can become full of stagnant blood and metabolic wastes that are not being properly removed by the now-inhibited lymph vessels due to the localized trauma — a ripple effect in traumatized muscle tissue — and nerve endings like proprioceptors become irritated by the lack of fluidity and pliability, potentially leading to pain and dysfunction. Examples of such tissue damage within skeletal muscles include trigger points and strains.

Natural Lymph Movement

In skeletal muscles, lymph vessels are compressed and lymph fluid is displaced from the muscle when it contracts. In visceral organs, lymph flow can be stimulated by the involuntary muscular actions of the gastrointestinal tract. In the heart, arterial pulsations can influence lymph movement. Contraction of the diaphragm affects lymph movement, too.

Smooth Muscle Functions

Smooth muscles are involuntary muscles associated with visceral organs. This form of muscle tissue wraps around the organ and initiates its movements from the exterior. The activities of smooth muscles are slow and rhythmic, and each visceral organ has its own sense of motion, called motility.

The digestive system has a unique form of involuntary contraction called peristalsis, a wave-like contraction that encourages material to move along the system's route. Its movement is slow, rhythmic and methodical, but peristalsis can become excessively slow and sluggish due to dehydration, poor diet and lack of exercise or medications. (See "Digestive System," page 60, for more information.)

The digestive system also contains tonic muscles, such as those in the various sphincters of the body, like the cardiac sphincter where the esophagus meets the stomach organ. Tonic muscles remain in a contracted state, only relaxing to allow materials to pass through the area.

DID YOU KNOW?

High-fiber diets and optimal hydration can stimulate natural peristalsis-like contractions in the colon.

Body Temperature Regulation

When muscles contract, they produce and release heat, which is important to maintain correct body temperature. When the body is cold, for example, it can rapidly contract (shiver) to produce heat. The actions of the circulatory and integumentary systems carry out the rest of this regulating process.

The body works best when internal temperatures stay within a relative range. When temperatures change, the body works to regulate this through combined efforts of the integumentary, circulatory and muscular systems.

How Cupping Affects the Muscular System

- **Promotes overall skeletal muscle health.** Manual therapies, such as massage and physical therapy, work continuously to encourage softness, pliability, hydration and overall loosening of these tissues when they are tense. Cups can create beneficial effects with negative pressure. Cupping encourages blood flow within the muscles, enhances the expression of accumulated metabolic waste and lymph movement, lifts and stretches these tight muscle fibers and decompresses any pressure on nerves that may pass through the muscles. Fascial adhesions are encouraged to soften and manipulation is made more accessible.
- While manual therapies press into muscles and work across their fibers to create space and separation for greater blood flow, cupping **lifts the tissue to create space** while simultaneously pulling blood into the area.
- While manual therapies press into muscles and work along the length of their fibers to stretch and move metabolic wastes such as lactic acid through them, cupping **lifts and rolls along the length of the muscle**, immediately elongating the tissue while simultaneously purging metabolic waste.
- **Promotes lengthening of tight muscles.** Cupping can stimulate the proprioceptive nerve endings within the muscles. Whenever a muscle is tight, there is nerve activity that is keeping it in a state of contraction. Cupping can lift and stretch the tissue rather than press into it, which tricks the contracted muscle into thinking it is lengthening and therefore stimulates a relaxation response.
- **Encourages lymph movement.** While cups can help with overall fluid functions involving lymph in muscle tissue, a cup can also "wring out" old, stagnant lymph from muscles. This is true in most cases, from repetitive motion injuries and traumatic accidents to stress and immobility (such as being bedridden).
- **Stimulates peristalsis.** Focusing on the large intestine, peristalsis can be stimulated with slow, rhythmic applications of cupping over the appropriate abdominal regions. The negative pressure can simulate the expansion that occurs during peristalsis and encourage this involuntary movement toward optimal colon function.
- **Supports body temperature regulation.** Muscles naturally work to regulate body temperatures. Cupping can help draw this heat to surface tissues for removal by both the pulling of the negative pressure as well as the increase in vasodilation.
- **Promotes muscle recovery.** For more information on muscle recovery, see "Athletic Performance and Cupping," page 230.

SKELETAL SYSTEM

ANATOMY

The skeletal system is composed of bones, cartilage, ligaments and joints.

FUNCTIONS

- Supports the body with its bony framework.
- Protects the body's vital organs.
- Provides leverage through muscle attachments.
- Houses hemopoiesis (forming of blood cells) in the marrow of the bones.
- Bones serve as a reservoir for necessary fats and minerals until the body needs them.

What Is Periosteum?

Bones are made up of various mineralized osseous (bony) tissues and are coated by periosteum. Periosteum is a sheath of dense vascular connective tissue that wraps around the bone and penetrates into it. It contains many blood and lymph vessels, nerves and various bone-growing cells (osteoblasts), and is the site where tendons and ligaments attach.

Formation of a Joint

The articulating surfaces of bones involved in joints have cartilage instead of periosteum. Cartilage is a form of connective tissue that offers both cushioning and protection from bones rubbing against each other. The more mobile joints of the body (diarthrosis) are composed of these cartilage-covered ends of bones, as well as ligaments, joint capsules and synovial membranes filled with fluids. Some diarthrodial joints also contain bursae (for example, the ischial tuberosity bursa located deep inside the hip joint), another fluid-filled body that offers additional cushioning within a joint where tendons may rub over bony surfaces.

Anatomy FYI

Synovial fluid is a gelatinous material that provides both nutrition and lubrication to highly mobile diarthrodial joints.

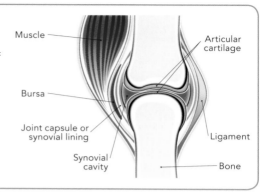
Inflammation in Joints

Inflammation is a leading cause of painful joint conditions. Joint inflammation creates stiff and painful sensations, often limiting the range of motion. Diarthrodial "synovial" joints, such as the shoulder joint, contain synovial fluid and joint capsules — they can become irritated and inflamed, leading to various painful inflammatory conditions like arthritis or osteoarthritis or other inflammatory conditions, such as frozen shoulder. Amphiarthrodial joints like the vertebrae can also have inflammation, but it is typically found on the surface of the vertebrae due to degeneration of the intervertebral discs. Bursitis is inflammation within bursae structures, such as the hip joint. Direct inflammation of the periosteum, known as periostitis, can be caused by overuse or injury — the most common example is shin splints — and can create a lot of localized pain.

Sometimes inflammation can be an autoimmune dysfunction that mistakenly attacks the body's own healthy tissue and creates inflammation within a joint, such as with rheumatoid arthritis. Inflammation is a major contributing factor to countless pathologies all over the body, not just within joints. (See Chapter 10: "Advanced Applications" for more information.)

How Cupping Affects the Skeletal System

- **Relieves inflammation.** If a joint is acutely inflamed, working more proximal areas (if on a limb, the area that is closer to the torso) and regional cupping can support the healing process. More chronic inflammations respond greatly to cupping directly over the area, due to the ability to encourage vasodilation while simultaneously drawing inflammation to the surface lymphatic system for disposal. (See "Working with Inflammation" in Chapter 10 for more information.)
- **Works with limited range of motion.** Cups can offer tissue hydration and lift up those structures that may be restricting movements within various joints of the body. Strategic placement of stationary cups around these inhibited joints may offer an improvement in overall joint flexibility and, ultimately, improved mobility. (See Chapter 8 for some basic applications to certain joints, such as the shoulder or knee.)

RESPIRATORY SYSTEM

ANATOMY

The respiratory system is composed of the nose and nasal cavity, pharynx, larynx, trachea, bronchi, bronchioles, alveoli, lungs and the respiratory diaphragm.

FUNCTIONS

- Exchanges oxygen and carbon dioxide during respiration.
- Detects smell through the nose and nasal cavity.
- Produces speech when wind from the lungs passes over folds in the larynx (voice box).
- Regulates pH (levels of acidity in the body) by controlling how much carbon dioxide the body releases.

The Breathing Mechanism

Respiration is an involuntary function of the body, yet it can be voluntarily influenced, for example, when taking a deep breath or holding your breath. The act of breathing is considered a vital bodily function since the rest of the body could not exist without it. Inspiration, or inhalation, takes oxygen into the body, while expiration, or exhalation, removes carbon dioxide. Every cell in our bodies need oxygen to survive — without it, cells can die and life would quickly cease to exist.

How Do We Get Oxygen?

When we breathe in, air travels into the lungs, where millions of tiny receptacles, called alveoli, are ready to receive oxygen. The job of the alveoli is to take in oxygen and, through tissue respiration, supply this oxygen to the capillaries that surround them, thereby allowing the oxygen to enter the bloodstream. From there, the capillaries take this oxygen–rich blood out to all the distal points of the body for distribution. The same process is reversed when veins deliver carbon dioxide–enriched blood back to the lungs. This process is how our bodies process oxygen and carbon dioxide exchange.

Anatomy FYI

Tissue respiration is the exchange of gases (oxygen, carbon dioxide) through a permeable membrane. This is how oxygen is extracted from air and put into blood circulation.

Mobility of Lung Tissues

The lungs are encased by slippery membranes called pleura, which are lubricated by pleural fluids. Any inflammation of the pleural fluids within this space, such as pleurisy, can be harmful. The outermost coating is called the pleural lining and it directly connects to the inside of the rib cage. There are two *pleura* in the thoracic cavity: one serves to enclose the lungs, while the other contains the entire thoracic cavity. Between the two there is *pleural fluid*, which lubricates movements, inhibiting any friction. During respiration, the lungs slide up and down as well as expand and contract, and both pleura and their fluids tremendously support this activity.

The Muscles of Breathing

The primary muscle responsible for respiration is the diaphragm, a large, flat muscle that divides the torso in half — the lungs and heart are above it, inside the thoracic cavity, and the rest of the visceral organs are below it in the abdominal cavity. The only openings in this large muscle are for the esophagus to enter the stomach and for the descending aorta to distribute blood from the heart to the lower body and the inferior vena cava (or large vein) to return blood from the lower body to the heart. The lungs rest directly on top of the diaphragm and move together through every breath.

Anatomy FYI

The *diaphragm* attaches to the spine, the xiphoid process (the bony prominence in the front of the body, at the base of sternum) and the entire ring of the 6th rib cage line.

When the diaphragm contracts, it lowers and allows for the lungs to expand and take in air — inhalation. When it relaxes, the diaphragm rises and supports the removal of air — exhalation.

While the diaphragm does most of the work, sometimes breathing can become labored or challenged (for example, bronchitis, shallow breathing) and some muscles are recruited to assist in the process. These muscles are called accessory muscles. Those that assist inhalation are the sternocleidomastoid, scalenes (both are in the front of the neck) and the pectoralis minor (located in the upper chest region, attaching to ribs and the acromion process, a bony process on the shoulder blade). The internal intercostals (the muscles between the ribs) and the abdominal muscles also help with expiration. These muscles already serve primary skeletal muscle movements, and they can be easily fatigued by this "double duty" when required to help.

Getting the Phlegm Out

The mucus that is coughed out of the respiratory tract is called phlegm. Mucus serves the important function of trapping any foreign substances, such as viruses, and removing them from the body. Once the mucus traps these substances, the cilia in the respiratory tract — those tiny hair-like fibers that move in a rhythmic motion — work to remove it. When there is an excess of mucus, the mucociliary escalator becomes overloaded and its performance lags.

Anatomy FYI

The *mucociliary escalator* is the name for the combined effort of mucus and cilia to remove unwanted materials from the respiratory tract.

How Cupping Affects the Respiratory System

- **Assists in coughing.** Coughing is a natural bodily function necessary to clear the respiratory tract, and cupping can help this process. Quick applications of cupping can help loosen mucus and stimulate the expectorant action of the mucociliary escalator when there is an excessive production of mucus. The flash cupping technique is an effective application to help clear a cough.
- **Addresses lung tissues.** Cups are known to lift and stretch tissue. Stronger cupping can reach as deep as 4 inches (10 cm) into the body, so there can be some impressive penetrating effects. Applying cups over the lung region can add a little lift and gentle expansion to all the tissues directly below the cup: the intercostal muscles, the ribs, the pleura, potentially even the lungs themselves. Think of the suction pump-like effect of stimulated microcirculation, too. Any surface tissue cupping can in turn stimulate all the deeper tissues they connect to in that area of the body. Such applications along the back over the lungs not only encourage the strength of local circulation and penetration into the body, but also stimulate various local lung points along the spine.
- **Helps remove excessive heat.** Cups are major vasodilators, and when combining this widening of blood vessels with the pulling action of negative pressure, cupping helps pull out any heat that may be trapped in the body. Inflammation can occur when the inflammatory response is triggered (for example, bronchitis) or with certain chronic conditions (such as asthma).
- **Stretches breathing muscles**. All the muscles involved in breathing — primary or accessory — can benefit from the relief cupping offers. Moving cups over the entire rib cage region brings openness to the intercostal muscles and diaphragm, which are naturally in a condensed environment.

DIGESTIVE SYSTEM

ANATOMY

The digestive system is composed of the teeth, tongue, gastrointestinal tract and related accessory organs (liver, gallbladder, pancreas and salivary glands).

FUNCTIONS

- **To ingest**, the process of consuming foods and liquids.
- **To digest**, the process of breaking down food.
- **To absorb**, the process of taking digested materials into the body systems.
- **To defecate**, the process of eliminating waste materials from the body.

The Gastrointestinal Tract

The gastrointestinal, or GI, tract is one continuous line from the mouth to the anus. Also known as the alimentary canal, there are many organs (both primary and accessory) along this path, as well as processes that are responsible for all the functions of the digestive system.

From Start to Finish

The mouth takes in food, breaks it down and sends it along into the esophagus, where it meets the stomach organ at the cardiac sphincter. The sphincter muscles relax and allow food to enter the stomach, where digestive acids further the digestive process and minimal absorption begins. The material then leaves the stomach through the pyloric sphincter and enters the small intestine, where most nutrients are extracted, absorbed into the intestinal walls, and taken into the blood and lymph vessels for dispersal around the body accordingly. The remaining materials pass through the ileocecal valve and into the large intestine, where a very small amount of remaining nutrients are extracted and absorbed. All the waste that remains is formed into fecal matter, which the colon removes from the body through the anus.

Anatomy FYI

A *sphincter* is a ring of tonic muscle tissue that controls materials moving from one part of the digestive tract to the next. Examples include:

- *Cardiac sphincter:* connects esophagus to stomach
- *Pyloric sphincter:* connects stomach to small intestine
- *Ileocecal valve:* connects small intestine to large intestine

Muscle Movements within the GI Tract

Two types of muscular contractions take place in this system: tonic and peristaltic contractions.

Tonic contractions occur at the sphincter junctions between the organs. This muscle tissue contracts to retain separation between organs and relaxes to allow materials to pass through. If this function is challenged, the valves can become slack and dysfunctional.

Peristaltic contractions are a specialized type of slow, rhythmic contraction that moves food materials along the entire GI tract. This subtle movement (peristalsis) requires hydration and supple tissue for proper performance.

Healthy Colon Movements

The large intestine is where peristalsis can become most challenged. Waste materials gather in little pockets within the colon wall — known as haustra — and are propelled along each section of the colon by its soft muscle contractions. If the colon's function becomes challenged — whether by dehydration, side effects of medications, low-fiber diets or inactivity — this movement slows down and waste material gets backed up and ultimately hinders the entire system's output. The most notable sign of this is constipation.

Visceral Organ Health

The digestive system also includes accessory organs, such as the liver, gallbladder and pancreas. Each of these organs supports digestion with various secretions (for example, bile) and filtration processes, such as filtering blood. The liver has many functions, as well as supporting overall body detoxification. These organs are all densely covered with blood and lymph capillaries.

DID YOU KNOW?

The liver is the largest *internal organ* in the body. The skin is the largest *organ system* of the body.

How Cupping Affects the Digestive System

- **Influences tonic muscular activity.** The lift and stretch of a cup can offer some stretch and relaxation to these small rings of muscles that can in turn improve their overall tone. It is most important to have an excellent knowledge of anatomy to use cups over these areas. The easiest place to use cups is over the cardiac sphincter for treatment of acid reflux.
- **Stimulates peristalsis.** The easiest access point to apply cups is for the colon. The lifting and stretching of cups make this an effective technique to stimulate smooth muscle movements in this region. Cups enhance the natural stretch of the colon walls, loosening material that may be stuck in the haustra. These applications should be slow and rhythmic, mimicking the body's natural function.
- **Promotes overall abdominal health.** The abdominal cavity has a high concentration of blood and lymph vessels, so encouraging gentle lymphatic movements here can stimulate the general circulation associated with all the organs contained in this area.

ANATOMY

The nervous system is composed of the brain, spinal cord, meninges (membranes that protect the brain and spinal cord), cerebrospinal fluid, peripheral nervous system (divided into somatic and autonomic) and special sense organs (ears and eyes).

FUNCTIONS

- Receives input from the body's sensory receptors by detecting changes such as pressure, temperature and motion, both inside and outside of the body.
- Interprets and integrates all stimuli to elicit an appropriate response.
- Initiates motor output like muscular contractions and glandular secretions.
- Is responsible for mental processes such as thought and memory functions, as well as emotional responses, such as anger and anxiety.

Bodily Functions and the Central Nervous System

The central nervous system (CNS) is the foundation of all our bodily functions, and the workings of this system are both incredibly complex and vital to our existence. Without it, we would not live. The brain and spinal cord are the most central units of this system and are protected by the meninges, skull and spinal column. From there, the peripheral nervous system branches out into all regions of the body to both collect and deliver sensory information. Think of the peripheral nervous system as a two-way highway: information is constantly coming and going via the same route.

Cells of the CNS

The most basic cells of the central nervous system are neurons, which interpret and respond to all the body's stimuli. Neurons are protected by neuroglia (or glia), which are a form of connective tissue. These two combine to create the basic structure of the nervous tissues that initiate chemical reactions throughout the body, such as the release of neurotransmitters to target areas. Optimal nervous tissue performance requires healthy space within the layers of soft tissue through which various nerves are found and travel.

How Nerve Cells Transmit Information

Individual nerve cells connect at synapses — fluid-filled spaces between the cells that are capable of transmitting the information carried by the system from one cell to the next. Neurotransmitters are various chemicals located adjacent to these synapses and can be released into the system when a neuron responds to a stimulus. Nerve cells have various responses, which in turn decide what chemical should be released into circulation. A few examples of neurotransmitters include acetylcholine (for muscle contraction), histamine (for vasodilation) and serotonin (for mood and sleep regulation).

Nerve Tissues

Nerves are a group of organized nervous tissues that carry information in and out of the central nervous system and are responsible for conducting all the body's actions. Nerves come together and form various nerve tracts (such as the median nerve) to address various tissues of the body. A large grouping of these nerves, usually closer to the central line of the body, is called a plexus (for example, the brachial plexus of the upper extremity).

The Peripheral Nervous System

The nerves of the peripheral nervous system extend directly out from the brain and spinal cord and are divided into two sections, the somatic and autonomic nervous systems.

Safety Point

· ·

The vagus nerve is most superficially exposed in the anterior triangle of the neck. (See "Endangerment Sites," page 92, for more information.)

The somatic nervous system is considered the "voluntary" part of the peripheral nervous system, controls bodily functions like skeletal muscle activities and can be further divided into two segments, cranial and spinal nerves.

The cranial nerves come straight from the brain and mostly control actions of the head, neck and shoulders. The vagus nerve is the longest cranial nerve and governs some of the head's activities (hearing, speaking) as well as extending into the torso to innervate the organs of the torso and abdomen.

The spinal nerves come out of the spine and weave their way through joints, muscles and all varieties of connective tissues to reach their destinations. The largest and longest spinal nerve is the sciatic nerve, which innervates the entire lower extremity. Maintaining appropriate space around these nerves is imperative for optimal performance of many bodily functions.

The autonomic nervous system governs the involuntary, non–thought–controlled actions of the body, including organ functions, gland secretions and general circulation, and can be further divided into the sympathetic and parasympathetic nervous systems.

The sympathetic and parasympathetic nervous systems work in a closely complementary manner to maintain balance within the body. When one system is stimulated, the other relaxes. A good example of how they work together is the body's fight-or-flight response. When stress occurs, the sympathetic nervous system is stimulated and will initiate the proper internal responses to get the body out of the stressful situation (release adrenaline, fire up the heart rate, speed up breathing) while the parasympathetic nervous system rests. When the body is not in a stressful mode, the sympathetic nervous system rests and the parasympathetic system performs more tranquil activities, such as releasing serotonin and dopamine for rest and relaxation as well as stimulating organ functions like digestion. Both systems conserve their own energy when not needed, and they support each other's vital function. This balancing act is the ultimate example of homeostasis.

Sensory Receptors

The end points of the peripheral nerves, where information is received and transmitted to the brain to initiate an appropriate response, are called sensory receptors. As indicated in the previous sections on the integumentary and muscular systems, these receptors are located all over the body. There is also quite a variety of these sense-detecting organs. Some respond to all the five senses (touch, sight, smell, taste and hearing); some respond to chemical changes in the blood (chemoreceptors); others respond specifically to muscle tension and activities (proprioceptors and muscle spindles); while still others are specifically designed to respond to pain (nociceptors).

Here's how nerve endings and sensory organs can work: If a therapeutic application is too deep, relevant nerve endings will trigger an alarm to the brain. The body will respond accordingly, whether with verbal reaction (telling the therapist that's too much pressure) or creating a wincing reaction in the body to protect the area. If an area of the body is locked in a state of hyper-contracture (for example, with torticollis, involving painful neck spasms), the body will continue a vicious cycle of nerve-ending responses to the pain but cannot relax it on its own.

How Cupping Affects the Central Nervous System

- **Provides decompressive therapy.** With negative pressure, cups offer decompression wherever they are applied. Light suction pressure over sensory receptors in the skin promotes relaxation, while deeper pressure addresses muscular compression (such as sciatica). The lift and stretch of cupping helps soften any tissue that may be putting pressure on nerves or tight muscles triggering pain. Whether specific (such as tracking the sciatic nerve down the leg) or general (such as cupping along the sides of the spine to affect all the peripheral nerves for relaxation), cups create space and relax nervous tissue.
- **Promotes relaxation.** Consider the nerve endings located all over the body. Non-aggressive cupping has a universally calming effect on the entire central nervous system due to its relaxing effect on all sensory receptors. Light massage strokes, often called nerve strokes, can promote relaxation from the calming response it evokes in the central nervous system, while soothing cupping applications can induce deep relaxation.
- **Addresses nervous system conditions.** Nervous tissue is involved in a wide range of pain, dysfunction and pathologies. By providing decompressive therapy, cupping can help alleviate primary contributing factors of some conditions (such as headaches) and provide relief to symptoms of other more complicated conditions (for example, soften tight muscles and relieve spasms associated with cerebral palsy).

ANATOMY

The urinary system is composed of the kidneys, ureters, urinary bladder and urethra.

FUNCTIONS

- Eliminates metabolic waste.
- Adjusts pH and chemical composition of blood.
- Controls blood volume and fluid balance.
- Monitors blood pressure.
- Maintains homeostasis due to the many chemical balances performed within the system.

Blood Filtration and Balances

The kidneys work to keep bodily fluid levels balanced, as well as support blood filtration through different processes than those that occur in the circulatory system or the liver. Just as the lymphvascular system works to filter fluids in the interstitial spaces, so too a similar process occurs in the kidneys. The kidneys are supplied by renal arteries, which carry oxygen-rich blood into the organ to be filtered, helping maintain fluid levels of the body. If there is an excess of fluid volume, it can lead to edema.

The kidneys also work to keep fluid levels balanced, both chemically and by volume. They help to regulate levels of acidity by releasing glucose into the blood when necessary, support waste removal of substances like hydrogen (through urination), which may have altered blood, and monitor blood pressure. If blood pressure changes, they can excrete certain chemicals into the circulatory system to promote vasoconstriction, which decreases the diameter of blood vessels, resulting in slower circulation.

How Cupping Affects the Urinary System

- **Helps with urinary retention.** Remember, cups promote the movement of fluids. Gentle cupping to encourage lymphatic movements within the midsection of the body (lower back and abdomen) can both support the vital functions of the kidneys and directly affect the fluids that may be retained within the urinary system.
- **Exercise caution when cupping over the kidney region.** Because of the key role the kidneys play in maintaining overall healthy fluid balance, they should be protected and encouraged to maintain their work optimally without any interruption. Any excessive cupping over these organs could alter their functions and potentially damage their anatomical points of attachment. (See Chapter 5: "Safe Cupping" for more information.)

REPRODUCTIVE SYSTEM

ANATOMY

The female reproductive system is composed of the ovaries, fallopian tubes, ova, uterus and vagina. The male system includes the testes, sperm ducts, sperm, penis and urethra.

FUNCTIONS

- To reproduce; that is, produce and release bodily materials (for example, sperm, ova) necessary for conception.
- To assist the process of reproduction by supporting pregnancy.

A Healthy Internal Environment

The uterus regularly cycles through bodily tissues (menstruation) preparing for possible conception, and is the space in a woman's body where a baby is contained during pregnancy. When pregnancy occurs, the abdomen, lower back and pelvis work to create the best space possible for a healthy pregnancy — the body creates attachment sites to secure the baby, stabilizes fluids to support and cushion its development, and generally adjusts to accommodate all these processes.

IRREGULAR MENSTRUAL CYCLES

"Regular" menstrual cycles vary from person to person, but they generally occur approximately once a month. Irregularities in the cycle can occur for many reasons: stress, trauma, scar tissue, tight muscles, medications, eating disorders, endometriosis, ovarian cysts and a whole range of potential dysfunction or diseases.

PELVIS TISSUE RESTRICTIONS

Just like the rest of the body, the female reproductive system is made up of various soft tissues and is vulnerable to adhesions, tightness and restricted circulation. In the case of endometriosis, for example, endometrial tissue grows outside the uterus, which can cause irritation to surrounding tissues as well as pain and inflammation.

How Cupping Affects the Reproductive System

- **Promotes regional softening.** Using cups regularly to encourage general lymphatic drainage in the midsection (low back, hips, abdomen) or working to address any adhesions in the lower back and sacral region can help regulate menstruation and promote general regional comfort.
- **Relieves stress.** Irregular cycles can also be caused by excessive stress or traumatic experiences. If so, consider soothing applications of cups to promote overall stress relief and allow the body to return to its regular functions.

ENDOCRINE SYSTEM

While the central nervous system provides the primary support for bodily functions, the endocrine system is just as important for regulating functions and body chemistry. Its functions are stimulated by the autonomic nervous system, the part of the nervous system that controls bodily functions that are largely involuntary, such as breathing and digestive.

ANATOMY

The endocrine system is made up of completely internal glands (ductless glands) and their respective hormones.

FUNCTIONS

Produces and secretes hormones that:

- Regulate body functions (growth, metabolism, internal chemistry balances).
- Stabilize the body during times of stress (trauma, emotional stress, dehydration, starvation, etc.).
- Support the reproductive process.

How Cupping Affects the Endocrine System

Because of their effect on the circulatory system, cups can help distribute hormones. The endocrine glands are surrounded by a concentration of capillaries. The hormones enter the capillaries and join the bloodstream, traveling throughout the body to arrive at their targeted locations. Cups can help with optimal distribution of these hormones because they encourage blood circulation throughout the body.

EXOCRINE SYSTEM

ANATOMY

The entire exocrine system is made up of various glands: thyroid, salivary, sebaceous, sudoriferous, mammary, prostrate, lacrimal, mucous and the liver.

- salivary glands produce saliva in the mouth
- sebaceous glands produce sebum, an oily substance that lubricates the skin
- sudoriferous glands produce sweat
- mammary glands produce breast milk
- prostate glands produce semen
- lacrimal glands produce tears in the eyes
- mucous glands produce mucous in the various mucosal lined cavities, like the nasal cavity

FUNCTIONS

Produces secretions that go directly to target locations or exit the body (sweat, breast milk, saliva, bile from the liver, etc.).

How Cupping Affects the Exocrine System

Cups help influence fluid movements and increase overall circulation, from the sudoriferous glands located in the integumentary system to the liver's bile production to the mammary gland secretions within breast tissue.

PART 2
USING CUPS IN BODYWORK THERAPY

CHAPTER 4
Assessing the Skin After Treatment

MARKS WITH THERAPEUTIC CUPPING

CUPPING 101

Cupping marks can occur anywhere on the body, with any application. This chapter will elaborate on locations and techniques that are more likely to yield cupping marks.

When a cupping treatment leaves markings, the recipient might be alarmed by the skin's reaction. Understandably, they may have associated the markings with a procedure that may not have been carried out properly and expect to experience some form of pain. With cupping, however, marks are simply a sign in most cases that there has been a significant therapeutic release in the tissue. While lighter applications for lymphatic drainage or gentle moving cups should not mark the tissue, stationary cups or stronger moving cups may create marks. The type of mark (color, texture, temperature of the tissue) can offer some insight on what is happening below the surface.

Marks versus Bruises

While cupping marks are often referred to as bruises, there are definite differences between the two. One of the main differences is that bruises hurt when you touch them, whereas marks do not. Bruising can happen when the suction in cups is too strong or if cups are attached to the skin for too long. A bruise signifies trauma to the tissue, broken capillaries and blood pooling; similarly, cupping done incorrectly can result in purpura, petechia or ecchymosis, which can look like bruises.

Anatomy FYI

Contusions and *bruises* occur with a traumatic contact to the body. *Purpura* is purple blood spots from small capillaries bursting and blood pooling under the skin. This can occur in the skin, muscles and organs. *Petechia* is pinpoint-sized blood spots from broken small capillaries in the skin. *Ecchymosis* is the same blood-pooling as petechia but larger in diameter.

Why Marks Appear

When cups are applied, the vacuum pull can release interstitial debris (old blood, medications, foreign substances) from within the various layers of soft tissue wherever it may have become embedded, and then draw it to the surface tissues just under the skin for disposal; the marks are "visible" in the superficial layers of tissue where the lymphatic system exists. While marks may be sensitive when touched — similar to how you feel following a deep-tissue massage — they should never hurt. Furthermore, not every treatment will leave marks. If cups are used lightly to address superficial tissue, for example, there would typically be no markings afterwards. Cups can leave once rigid tissue soft, supple and hydrated without ever marking it. In fact, whether or not a treatment produces marks has no bearing on the treatment's effectiveness — marks should be considered an "added bonus" of release.

Once a mark is visible on the skin, it may last a few hours to a few days. How long it takes to disappear will vary on a number of contributing factors, including the degree of the marking. Darker and more profound markings may take longer to dissipate. Cupping should not be reapplied over existing marks so the body has a chance to fully process what has been released. Also, consider the health of the person's lymphatic system: the slower the system circulates, the longer the marks may take to disappear.

Initial and Subsequent Marks

Marking is more likely with initial applications than with subsequent cuppings. When cups are first applied, they can yield some impressive releases, as this method of therapeutic manipulation is entirely new to the body. However, a cup should never be applied only to produce marks. If this is the intention, chances are high that bruising, not marking, will occur. When therapeutic cupping is done correctly, the body will gladly release any unwanted substances (for example, old blood) that are embedded within the layers of tissue.

Some people may get marks time and time again, however, typically for a few reasons. For one, if an area of injury is reinjured after cupping was used in the recovery process, then cup marks can show up again. We see this with repetitive motion injuries, as in a baseball

DID YOU KNOW?

What's the Difference?
Cupping marks
- Are a response to interstitial debris being released during some cupping applications.
- May be sensitive, but should not be painful to touch.
- Will simply fade away; they do not change in color like a bruise does.

Bruises
- Are a response to an injury.
- Are painful when touched.
- Will fade and change in color or in demarcation as the traumatized blood loses oxygen (red and blue) and then is dissolved in the lymphatic system (yellow or brown).

CUPPING 101

A body's reaction to cupping will vary tremendously due to variations in diet, hydration, circulation, exercise and medical regimens. For this reason, markings need to be assessed according to the particular person receiving treatment, rather than assuming that any two marks are the same.

pitcher's shoulder. Every time an area is injured, stagnant blood will surface when cupped.

Also, areas of deeper stagnations or restrictions (for example, in the deeper layers of tissue in the gluteal region, such as those associated with sciatica) will respond cumulatively to cupping. In such instances, the surface tissues may produce marks at first in the process of releasing whatever material was more superficial (for example, the material the body is naturally trying to expel on its own over the site of stagnation). Once this release occurs, subsequent applications of cupping will cause the deeper levels of stagnations to rise and eventually be released. The body has quite an impressive method of burying material in its intricate layers of tissues. In its own time, the body tries to release these materials, and cups are powerful enablers of this process — think of cups as having the ability to slowly dredge up these substances rather than abruptly yank them out of the body.

Whether cupping leaves a lasting mark or reveals stagnation in the tissue without making a mark, consider a cup to be a "looking glass" into the body, revealing what issues may lie underneath the surface.

COLORS, TEMPERATURES AND TEXTURES

While there is no scientific research on what the different colors and textures of cupping marks mean, however, there is anecdotal proof of efficacy from consistent results. Remember, these marks are *not bruises* and any interpretations of what they mean should be done mindfully and with respect to the body from which they arose — different people will all have different marks.

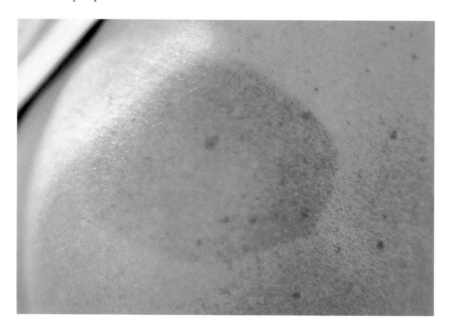

Colors

Light red or pink speckling: New, more superficial stagnations and restrictions are being released. This coloration may also signify the person is experiencing an acute condition, a recent injury or a current stressor, such as a marital breakup, during the time of treatment. Red and pink speckling is generally limited to the more superficial dermis or musculature.

Dark red or purple: Older, deeper stagnations are being released. This coloration can indicate a site of surgery, an intense illness or a long-term stressor, or an old injury, such as a deep bruise from falling on a hip years earlier where the blood stagnation was never fully expelled to the lymphatic system under the many layers of tissue in this region (see Client Work #2, page 81).

Purple, raised: Thicker material, generally old blood deposits, is being released. These marks can be palpated with the fingertips, using the lightest of touch to feel material that is located just under the skin but above the musculature and feel slightly raised. These deposits surface as soon as the vasodilation and vacuum are introduced, usually preceded by red speckling. Consider this a welcome release of old materials, most likely blood from old injuries or surgeries. As this is a powerful release, discontinue using cups for that session. Furthermore, it is strongly advised to encourage some lymphatic drainage (whether with hands or using cups lightly) so the waste material being released can be directed toward ultimate disposal via the lymphatic system.

When cupping is done incorrectly or too aggressively, dark purple balls like purpura are considered trauma to the tissue. While it can be difficult to differentiate between purple marks and bruises, remember that if cupping was done properly and there is no pain associated with the mark, this is a positive release.

Gray: This color most likely signifies the release of smoke, either first-hand or second-hand (second-hand is usually accompanied by a yellow hue to the area). Remember that the skin is a permeable barrier and smoke can easily invade the body, manifesting as gray-colored interstitial debris. Similarly, any inhaled smoke can enter into circulation via tissue respiration, eventually contributing to gray colored marks, too. We typically note this coloration in smokers, partners, children or other cohabitants of smokers, firefighters, coal miners or other persons with exposure to excessive amounts of smoke (such as bartenders where smoking is permitted or any environment where there is regular smoke exposure). These gray releases may be accompanied by the actual *smell* of smoke, too.

DID YOU KNOW?

In an essay, world-renowned cupping practitioner Bruce Bentley recounts an experience that occurred more than 20 years ago when Barry Cooper, the head massage therapist at the Australian Institute of Sport (AIS), was using cups to treat an athlete. When a dark cupping marking surfaced, Cooper immediately extracted a tissue sample and sent it off to a laboratory for testing. The results confirmed that it was the athlete's own old blood. This was one of the first pieces of science-based evidence to suggest that cupping could draw up these deposits.

Evaluate the Person, Not Just the Mark

Remember, marks should be evaluated according to the *person* in whom they surface. If a color surfaces, ask these types of questions:

- Have you ever been injured in the area where the cupping mark appeared?
- Have you ever had surgery?
- Do you have any scar tissue?
- Do you (or have you ever) smoked?
- Have you ever been exposed to toxic chemicals, such as pesticides?

For one individual, a yellow marking can signify a medication — such as a yellow syrup — they used to take regularly (and *tasted* when the color surfaced), while another person may have yellow coloring appear around surgical sites (like cesarean or C-section scars). One person may show green colors around a site of amputation and the related surgical medications, while another may present green colors around an area of the body that has been topically exposed to chemical fumes. These examples have all been seen in practice.

Working with Tissue Marks

Marks can happen at any time and you may continue working with cups even when they appear. If a lot of marking occurs, however, consider it an indication of some significant releases and consider the cupping finished for that session. Sometimes this can be 5 minutes, sometimes 20. What is most important is to be sure that the person receiving cupping isn't in pain afterwards and that they feel comfortable with any further applied therapy. While some people may want it "all out now" (such requests are made frequently!), it is important to understand that the body works toward optimal balance — homeostasis — logically, and making alterations too quickly can cause some pretty serious reactions. Too much cup work can cause swelling, pain, nerve irritation and bruising, among other potential problems.

Yellow: More like a hue to the tissue rather than a lasting mark, yellow is most likely lymph that was not moving through an area (around scars) or areas of congestion (such as sinus congestion). Yellow may also signify old medications that haven't been disposed of by the body's own methods, and the person may actually report *tasting* old medications (for example, bronchial syrups) or nicotine (first-hand or second-hand smoke) that was not disposed of by the lymphatic system and has remained in the interstitial spaces.

White/lack of color: Seeing a lack of coloring often signifies a deficiency, whether due to poor blood circulation within an area (for example, ischemic [See Anatomy FYI, below] muscles not receiving proper blood flow) or if a person is deficient in energy (for example, depression).

Green: While rare, seeing such coloration signifies the release of old medications (such as anesthesia) or toxins that remained in the system, either as the result of a surgery years earlier or from external pathogens (exposure to chemicals) such as pesticides, toxic inhalants or air pollution.

Anatomy FYI

Ischemia is a term used to define an area lacking sufficient blood supply. A tight, restricted muscle is *ischemic. Hyperemia* is a term used to define an increase in blood supply to an area. After a massage, tissue can look red due to its new *hyperemic* state.

Temperatures

While visible marks can tell a tale of release, so too can any changes in the surface temperature of skin. When preparing to apply cups, take note of the temperature of the skin. If the skin turns pink or red (not a marking but a change in color) and feels cool or hot when the cup is removed, lightly feel the surrounding, untreated area for comparison. When the temperature of the skin changes between the start and finish of a treatment but leaves no visible mark, this is also a type of cupping release. Here's what the temperatures signify:

Warm: When the cupped area is visibly pink and warm to the touch, this signifies a good increase of blood flow to the area, also known as hyperemia.

Hot: When the cupped area is visibly pink or red and significantly warmer than the surrounding tissue, it can be indicative of inflammation, such as bursitis or tendonitis, drawn to the surface.

As a permeable barrier, skin is exposed to outside elements, including cold air, wind, bad energies (from the people around us) or toxic substances — all of which can affect the temperature of skin.

Cold: When the cupped area is visibly pink or red yet cold to the touch, this is an anomaly that most practitioners define as an old restriction, likely from an old injury, being released. Logically, you would expect that any tissue being worked on and turning red would be warm to the touch, but that does not happen in this case. Cold could also signify that the body was at some point subjected to extremely cold temperatures within weeks of a cupping treatment — perhaps the body didn't have time to acclimatize to a different climate or experienced instances of sudden and extreme exposure to cold during a windy or blustery day. In these instances, cold on the skin following a cupping treatment can be a sign of a positive release.

Textures

Crackling, crunching or gristly sensations while moving cups: The sensation of these textures *through* a cup as you move it is normal, especially over areas of stagnant metabolic waste (such as lactic acid) or soft-tissue restrictions (such as the IT band). As with hands massaging an area to feel the texture in the tissue, cups can also detect textures that are not smooth. When there are restrictions in the IT band, for example, cups often detect crunchy textures as they move along the area.

Cup "sticking" while moving: If the cup is sliding around an area with a comfortable light-to-medium suction and it "sticks," the cup has identified an underlying area of restriction. To feel this sensation requires an awareness of your tactile perception while moving a cup; pay attention as you move the cup, comparing one section of tissue to the next. The slower the cup moves, the easier it is to feel this subtle difference in tension.

Safety Point

There will be some sticking as you slide along the mid- to lower back and over the kidneys, due to their superficially exposed anatomical position and their structural attachments located within this area. Remember, no strong or aggressive cupping should be done directly over the location of the kidneys; refer to Chapter 5: "Safe Cupping" for more information about working in this region.

ADHESIONS

Cups will "stick" as they move across an area where tissue is adhered. If structures are extra restricted, there may be visible indentations when the cup is placed over this area.

Optimally, the tissue should rise up like a dome when a cup is applied. This is true for soft and pliable tissues because they are well hydrated and not stuck together. However, when tissue is extra tight, restricted or bound down (such as the unseen tension over the shoulder blade), adhesions may be detected and offer insight into someone's discomfort. The ability to literally see the restriction can help identify the root cause of pain, which may not be discovered by other methods of assessment.

Adhesions are also a great tool for clinical documentation. If you happen to locate an adhesion that seems to be a major contributing factor to an individual's pain, say within the infraspinatus muscle (which is part of the rotator cuff muscle group on the scapula), note it and see how it responds in a future application.

Anatomy FYI

Adhesions are defined as any two anatomical surfaces stuck or growing together that do not naturally connect, usually due to injury or inflammation. This can be within muscles, connective tissues, visceral organs and even across body systems. For more information on how adhesions affect the body, see Chapter 2: "How Cupping Affects the Body."

Client Work

During treatment, as soon as the cup latches onto a stuck tissue, the person receiving the work will often acknowledge it as being "on the spot!" Indeed, the spot may be visible to the person applying the cups as an adhesion. In one case, a client who came in for treatment suffered lingering pain after shoulder surgery. While cupping around the entire joint, the cup latched onto an adhesion in the infraspinatus muscle. This discovery was exciting because it identified a significant restriction and we started to work this newly identified area to resolve the source of pain.

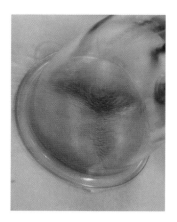

EXAMPLE OF ADHESION

This adhesion was not visible without cups. Here, the client complained of lower back discomforts and irregular menstrual cycle (her doctor told her she was premenopausal). When the cup was placed over the lumbosacral junction (see Anatomy FYI, below), the client immediately felt a connection into her lower abdomen, a sort of pulling from the back of her body. The cup was left on for a few minutes, removed, and then reapplied for another few minutes. A few days after her treatment, the client began her menstrual cycle. After many regular treatments, which also included abdominal work, the client's menstrual cycle became regular again.

Anatomy FYI

The *lumbosacral junction* is where the lumbar spine (base of spine) joins the sacrum (tailbone). Some nerves that innervate the abdomen pass through this region, known as the *sacral plexus*.

OTHER CONSIDERATIONS WITH TISSUE MARKS

Different areas of the body may mark more easily than others. This may be due to the thickness of the tissue or the degree of tension in certain areas. Wherever the surface tissue and skeletal bones are closer together, and hence the area between them is thinner, there is limited space to distribute or hide stagnation and cupping marks may easily occur.

Thinner areas include:

- over the neck
- over the scapula (e.g., rotator cuff muscles, trapezius, etc.)
- along the spine (e.g., erector spinae muscles)
- over any bony prominences or joints (e.g., tendonitis in the elbow or around the knee)

Thicker areas of anatomy can still reveal embedded stagnations, but not necessarily leave a mark that will remain for a few days.

Thicker areas include:

- the hips and gluteal region
- legs
- arms
- feet
- hands

Client Work #1

LASTING CUPPING MARKS

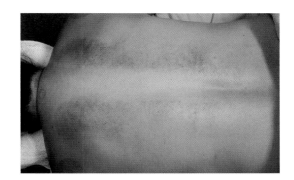

The client is very active and was complaining of overall back, neck and shoulder tension. While the client marks regularly and easily, she does not experience any pain. This coloring is normal and not bruising.

Client Work #2

DEEPER REGIONS OF ANATOMY

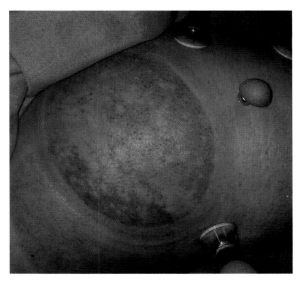

The client is in a prone position (lying face down) and cups were applied to the right gluteal region. During his first two treatments, there was faint, underlying congestion in the entire gluteal area but the cups left no marking. A third treatment showed a marble-like marking, but it did not leave a lasting cupping mark. A reddish purple color, particularly near the hip joint (the greater trochanter of the femur), where the tissue is less vascular at the attachments, along with white, or an absence of color, was prominent. It was discovered that the client had fallen on his right hip more than 10 years earlier. He had experienced chronic pain in the general gluteal and lower back area, especially on his right side. The treatment, done over a few sessions, has removed the majority of the client's pain.

CHAPTER 5

Safe Cupping

CONTRAINDICATIONS, SAFETY AND CONSIDERATIONS

In general, the same contraindications and safety considerations apply to working with cups as they do to massage, other bodywork or applied therapies. You would not attempt to manipulate an open wound during a massage, for example, so you would not apply a cup on it either.

As a point of reference, if it can be massaged, it can be cupped. In most cases, this is a good guideline; however, there are a few exceptions. One in particular is the case of varicose veins: you can gently glide over varicose veins with your hands, but absolutely no cups should be used over varicose veins. If you are uncertain about the safety or treatment of a particular condition with cups, it is probably best not to use them. Cupping could affect far too many pathologies that need to be noted, so be sure to evaluate the condition — that is, the person — and work accordingly.

Consider the effects cupping has on the body: cups lift, separate and stretch tissue. Cupping influences fluids — blood and lymph — around the body and releases toxins and waste products from different layers of tissue.

Safety Point

If it's difficult to decide whether or not to use cups, the world of bodywork typically refers to this statement: *When in doubt, refer out.* Whether you are a beginner or a highly trained practitioner, when the protocol is uncertain, consider referring a client to a practitioner who is better suited to deal with the issue.

CONTRAINDICATIONS

While cups can be applied to almost every body, there are situations when they should not be used or they should be applied with caution and control. In these situations, therapeutic cupping should **not** be used:

- Never use cups over open wounds.
- Never use cups when a person has deep vein thrombosis (DVT).
- Avoid using cups over any contagious skin conditions (chicken pox, herpes blisters) or topical irritants (poison ivy, unknown rash).
- Never apply cups directly on top of varicose veins; cups could cause further damage.
- Never apply cups directly over bulging or herniated discs, or any severely compromised joints, such as a sprained or dislocated knee.
- Avoid using cups directly on recent injuries such as bruises, sprains, strains or fractures. In general, wait *at least* 4 weeks before working directly over these areas unless otherwise instructed by the health-care provider attending to the injury. Bruises can be worked *gently* after about 14 days to help facilitate lymphatic clearing; the more severe the bruising, the gentler the work should be and the longer you should wait before applying cups. Less severe strains can be worked *gently* after *the initial pain* state has ended, as this may accelerate healing. Clinically trained practitioners may choose to work within different time parameters, but this is done at the professional's discretion.
- Avoid using cups directly over the belly button, as this is an open orifice into the body.

SAFETY

Cups can be used in various circumstances with some modifications. In the following situations, cups can be used safely by varying their applications to each individual scenario.

GENERAL

- Use caution when working in endangerment sites. (See "Endangerment Sites," page 92, for more information.)
- Begin with lighter suction for initial applications. It is important to increase suction *only* when it is comfortable and does not hurt. Cups should never hurt!

BODY AREAS

- Use lighter suction over any superficial vascular areas; see section regarding vascular considerations on page 88 for further information on this subject.
- To ensure proper lymph drainage, be sure to drain and clear more proximal regions of limbs (closer to the trunk) before working the distal areas (furthest from the trunk). For example, address the upper arms before the forearms and thighs before the lower legs; otherwise, you could overload or back up the lymphatic system (see Chapter 9: "Therapeutic Cupping for Lymphatic Drainage" for more information).
- Use caution when working in the abdomen. This area of the body houses many vital organs and the dermal covering is thinner than that of the back body. Any aggressive work done here could not only damage such crucial anatomy, but also easily inflame the adipose (fat) tissue in this region.
- Avoid sliding the cup over any raised moles or skin tags; cups could hurt or potentially tear tissue.
- Avoid scraping the cup over any bones, as this can be painful.

Anatomy FYI

Panniculus, also known as pannus, is the term for the subcutaneous adipose tissue located in the lower abdomen. *Panniculitis* is inflammation of this adipose tissue.

TARGET GROUPS

- **Working with children:** Use light to medium suction. The liver is not fully developed until about age 18, so be wary of any waste (for example, interstitial debris, metabolic waste like lactic acid) that may be released from excessive cupping as to not overload the liver's filtration processes. Younger tissue may also mark or bruise more easily. In general, the younger the tissue, the more lightly you should work. For example, I have had success with gently cupping a 4-month-old baby to treat colic.
- **Working with older clients:** Use light to medium suction. The thinner the skin, the more delicate the tissue's integrity, so be sure to use lighter suction. As we age, tissue loses elasticity and skin can loosen or sag. Exercise caution with stronger suctions or vigorous work if there are degenerative conditions like osteoporosis and degenerative disc disorder (when working along the spine) or if the client is taking a lot of medications.

COMMON HEALTH CONDITIONS AND ISSUES

- Use caution with anyone taking several medications. Consider the contraindications noted for each medication and adapt the therapy, if possible, during treatment.
- When working with eczema, psoriasis, atrophic dermatitis or other skin conditions, exercise caution when using cups over any compromised areas of tissue that appear inflamed, red, peeling or cracked.
- Avoid strong or excessive work on people taking blood thinners, which compromise the circulatory system — bruising and tissue damage can occur more easily.
- Use lighter suction if working on spider veins.
- Be cognizant that lipomas (benign tumors composed of fatty tissue), adipose deposits (tissue irregularities formed from fatty tissues) or any other tissue abnormalities vary widely in textures, sensitivities and composition. Some may be sensitive to bodywork, while others (such as some non-cellulite-related adipose deposits like those in a runner's quadriceps) may be cupped without discomfort and could even benefit from some simple cupping.
- Be cautious when using cups directly on top of any acne (pimples, blackheads), as you may pop them and express the contained fluids, leaving an open wound.
- Avoid working on new tattoos. Any tattoos older than at least 1 month can receive cupping with no potential risk of damaging the artwork or tattooed tissue, which is essentially wounded. The newer the tattoo, the lighter the suction and the lesser the time that should be applied to the area.

SPECIFIC MEDICAL CONDITIONS

- **Working with people with diabetes:** Cupping can be very beneficial for individuals with diabetes, but there are several considerations to note, in particular changes in blood sugar and skin condition that can affect treatment.
- **Working with oncology patients:** Cupping is possible, but it requires a specially trained practitioner with a thorough knowledge of the lymphatic system and oncology care.
- **Working with cysts:** If cystic tissue is present, be sure to evaluate the type of cyst before attempting to apply any cups. For example, a Baker's cyst — a bulge or cyst caused by fluid buildup in tissue behind the knee — affects the knee joint and surrounding structures. Cupping can help encourage fluid drainage from the joint area. A ganglion cyst, which is a fluid-filled sac that commonly occurs in the wrist area, should not be directly cupped because this could worsen the situation. Some forms of endometriosis can involve cystic tissue outside the uterus and can benefit from gentle abdominal and lower back cupping, while sebaceous cysts, cysts on the skin, can be gently cupped and encouraged to dissipate.

- **Working with joint replacements:** Cupping can be used here, but be mindful not to use excessive suction at the site of the replacement, especially if the individual is still experiencing sensitivity. The more recent the replacement, the less aggressive the cup work. The average wait time to use cups is 4 to 6 weeks after the surgical procedure.
- **Working post-surgery:** The average wait time is about 4 to 6 weeks before working with cups. If still not entirely certain, consider waiting longer before treatment or (preferably) get written consent or release from the individual's doctor.
- **Working with abdominal mesh:** Use extremely light suction over any surgically implanted abdominal mesh (from hernias or reconstructive surgeries) or avoid the area entirely. If anything, applications should be for light, lymphatic movement in the general area; the more compromised the area, the more it is recommended to avoid using cups entirely.
- **Working with injections:** Injection zones, whether cosmetic injections in the thin face tissue or cortisone shots in the deeper hip joint, should not be cupped. Wait a minimum of 30 days after injection to attempt *any* cupping. Even then, cups should never be strong and cupping should not be aggressive because you could dislodge the material and move it around the body.

    Some injected materials are intended for local circulation distribution, such as substances like prolotherapy, which is meant to stimulate the body's own inner inflammatory healing response; if choosing to use cups around this location, be sure that you are not trying to remove material from the intended site of application, rather that you can safely work close to the site without much limits on time. Other injection sites, like those for insulin, can be lightly cupped around the area, but be mindful of the person's sensitivity or avoid the region entirely until their own circulation process has distributed the substance.
- **Working on scar tissue:** Be cautious here, especially with new or keloid or hypertrophic (atypical scars that can be worsened if overstimulated) scars. (See "Scar Tissue and Cupping" in Chapter 10 for more information.)

CUPPING 101

Apply only the lightest of suction pressures over the area; consider what has been injected and the layer of tissue it was put into.

OTHER CONSIDERATIONS

Bodies vary, and so too will certain attributes that could affect cupping, such as excess hair or skin elasticity. Certain practices could also pose potential problems if the cupped area is exposed following treatment. Keep these factors in mind:

- **Avoid hot tubs, pools, steam treatments or saunas for a few hours after cupping.** The cups encourage vasodilation, which can alter the normal levels of heat and fluid exchange in the body, so increased exposure to heat too soon afterward could potentially cause swelling from the excessive movement of fluids. There is also a possibility for skin irritations, such as a rash, due to the increased exposure through the dilated vessels.

  If a heat treatment is desired (bodyworkers often apply heat to 'warm up' an area before manipulating it), chose to do so *before* any cupping; the tissue will naturally soften from the applied heat, perhaps allowing for a more comfortable and positively responsive cupping experience.

THERAPEUTIC THOUGHT: EPSOM SALT BATH

While I always encourage a warm Epsom salt bath after a massage, when a client receives cupping, I suggest they wait a few hours (at least 2) so their body tissues have the chance to settle. I also encourage them to drink plenty of water while in the bath to replenish the fluid that has moved to surface tissues.

- **Avoid cold temperatures, if possible, for a few hours after cupping.** Due to vasodilation and an overall openness of the tissue following cupping, cold temperatures can reach down to the core and shock the body's internal temperature and environment. If you live in a colder climate, make some attempts to keep warm after treatments, such as applying layers of clothing, wearing scarves and avoiding drafts and/or outdoor activity.

- **Limit tissue exposure post-treatment.** Again, vasodilation and the opening of tissue could make the body more susceptible to exterior hazards invading the internal environment, whether these hazards come from the surrounding environment (such as smoke, chemical fumes, etc.) or an energy source (such as another person's anger). Cover tissue, if possible, for an appropriate period of time (under clothing is fine) until the increased vasodilation has neutralized — a minimum of 2 hours and maximum overnight. If therapeutic cupping on an entire shoulder and back area leaves the tissue soft, pliable and red, for example, it is recommended to keep covered for at least 2 hours to allow vasodilation to settle. If full body cupping has been applied to mimic lymphatic drainage, the area can be left uncovered if necessary.

CUPPING 101

Cold is thought to be an invasive, pathogenic factor in Traditional Chinese Medicine. Any potential for the cold to invade the body is considered a pathway to sickness.

- **Avoid exercise for at least a few hours after using cups.** Muscles can be in an altered state (stretched, loosened) and exercises could be less effective or potentially cause damage. There are a few exceptions, however. If physical therapy is being employed along with cupping, perform only the exercises recommended under professional instruction, or for pre-event sports (whether days before or a same-day event, on-site work like that performed by athletic trainers) preparations that use cupping to loosen muscles, but keep in mind that cups should not be too strong or left on for too long. Be sure to gently introduce this work with practices — don't begin using cups on the day of an event — to see how the body responds.
- **Burns.** First- and second-degree burns can benefit greatly from cupping. Third-degree burns can be cupped and generally also respond well; however, they should be approached with caution and gentle initial suction. Cups should be applied only after tissue is fully healed and is approved for general massage and bodywork. The more compromised the skin, the longer this time period may be.
- **Excessive body hair.** People with heavy body hair may require more lotion or oil than normal to get cups to stick to the skin, and some might be too hairy to receive cups at all.
- **Loose skin.** This condition may pose a challenge. Be mindful not to use too much suction just to get a cup to adhere, since this can be painful. You could try using one hand to hold the loose skin taut as you slide the cup when you are trying to move it.

FURTHER GUIDELINES WITH SAFE CUPPING APPLICATIONS

While there are many items that give specific information on limitations and guidelines for using cups, there are certain conditions and physical elements (for example, endangerment areas) that require further evaluation, consideration and direction. For more information about specific cupping application or techniques referenced in the upcoming sections, see Chapter 7: "Using Cups in Treatment."

VASCULAR CONSIDERATIONS

- **Backs of hands and tops of feet:** Be careful when applying cups over superficial arteries and veins if it is possible to place cups on these surfaces (it may not be possible due to their bony composition).
- **Varicose veins:** Do not use cups directly on top of varicose veins; cups here could cause further damage. You can work proximal (closer to the torso when on a limb), close to and around but not directly on top of the vein.

- **Spider veins:** Lighter suction cups can be used directly over spider veins (dilated, superficial blood vessels that pool blood when damaged; challenged circulation can worsen them). If cups are used on a regular basis and address the entire region (for example, cups applied on the thigh if spider veins are on the outside of the thigh), there may be cumulative effects that reduce the appearance of spider veins by encouraging blood flow. See Chapter 3: "Therapeutic Benefits on the Body Systems" for more information on blood vessels in the circulatory system.
- **Superficial vascular areas:** Do not use strong suction wherever vascular bodies are more superficially exposed, such as the inside of the arms. This could cause damage to the vessels.

Anatomy FYI

While blood vessels can be superficially exposed anywhere, the most common areas are the anterior (inside) of forearm, inside of upper arm, back of hand, top of foot and temporal region (next to the eyes on the face).

CIRCULATORY CONSIDERATIONS

- **Working on the arms and legs:** Stationary cups have a strong influence on blood and lymph circulation, so use caution when placing them on the limbs for longer periods. When applying stationary cups, such as in the IT band, it is strongly advised to follow with an application of movements, either with cups or hands, that will encourage recirculation toward the torso.
- **Working on the neck:** The neck is a very delicate part of the body, so any stronger work should be done solely to the posterior aspect of the neck (behind the ears). Furthermore, the direction should be generally away from the head, whether side to side or toward the torso. (See "Endangerment Sites," page 92, for more information.)

Pathological Considerations

While there are far too many pathologies to list, there are two very common ailments that should be specifically addressed. Here, diabetes and cancer will be briefly covered, however, any pathology can be evaluated and analyzed to see if someone can receive cupping. See "Evaluation: Center on the Person, Not the Condition," page 94, for further information.

CUPPING AND DIABETES

Using therapeutic cupping on people with diabetes can yield great results, but certain precautions need to be acknowledged. When people have diabetes, their circulation is challenged and their sensitivity to touch can be more palpable, both of which may make the potential for working too aggressively more likely.

- **Changes in blood sugar.** Massage can lower blood sugar levels. Because cups enhance the body's exchange of fluids, it is advisable to check sugar levels before and after treatment. The more intense the condition, the stronger the advisory.
- **Sensitivity in the hands and feet.** Any neuropathy, in particular the nerve damage caused by diabetes, can cause extra sensitivity in the hands and feet. Cups can be used and are potentially quite beneficial, but work mindfully.
- **Avoid working on any severely damaged, necrotic tissue and never work on any open ulcerated tissue.** Cupping can help improve damaged tissue in the lower limbs, but this work should only be done by a trained professional. Any application's primary consideration is to stimulate overall circulation to the entire limb. The most distal (furthest from the torso) portion, such as the lower calf, is often the most damaged; working in this area should not be attempted until the more proximal regions, such as the thigh and upper calf, have experienced positive change.

THERAPEUTIC THOUGHT: WORKING WITH ULCERATED TISSUE ON LIMBS

In my experience, when using cups to promote overall tissue health where ulcerated tissue on distal limbs is a factor, treating the more proximal areas has a direct effect on the more distal areas. Only after the ulcerated tissue has closed and fully healed can any work be done over this tissue. Also keep in mind that this area can be very sensitive and painful if suction pressure is too strong. The lift-and-release technique with the lightest possible suction should be applied first in the most delicate region. Only after this is comfortable should any moving cups be attempted. Cumulative applications work best here. For more on cupping techniques, see Chapter 7.

CUPPING AND ONCOLOGY CARE

Cancer is a very complicated condition and it affects every patient differently. Massage and bodywork are approved when the timing is right, and this is usually dictated by the doctor administering the patient's care. Cancer survivors typically receive appropriate bodywork with little to no complications; however, keep these factors in mind when using cups on cancer patients.

- **No cupping work should be done while someone is in active chemotherapy or radiation.** Cups strongly affect the movement of fluids, and because medications being administered in the cancer treatment are meant to target specific areas of the body, cups should not be used during this time. Wait until at least 4 to 6 weeks after treatments are completed before using cups unless a doctor's written consent is given.
- **If unsure, do not use cups.** Oncology care is very complicated and details vary tremendously. Bodily tissue can be volatile or excessively damaged from the wide variety of illnesses and related procedures that surround such a disease. From surgical extractions and radiation to compromised lymphatic dysfunction or reconstruction (for example, mastectomy), cups could cause harm if used incorrectly. Be sure to contact a trained professional if any concerns about using cups exist.

THERAPEUTIC THOUGHT: HOSPICE CARE

I have worked on people going through final end-of-life care, and while it may seem contraindicated, I have received approval from their doctors. Healing touch is extremely therapeutic and cups can have the same effect as caring hands when used correctly.

Safety Point

Therapists who are specially trained in oncology care may choose to work outside the guidelines suggested here, but that is up to the professional's discretion. This book is meant to give universal information on safety.

Endangerment Sites

Anterior Triangle

Use *only* light suction and the lift-and-release technique across the entire front of the neck region, commonly called the anterior triangle. This general vicinity (in front of the ears, bilaterally) should be protected from any strong suction, stationary cups or gliding movements. Any suction that is too strong could possibly cause a tear in the vital blood vessels located here, which could potentially lead to a hemorrhagic stroke. Cups should only be worked down the neck, toward the trunk so they do not draw fluid into the head, potentially causing head congestion or a headache.

- The carotid artery (and all its branches), jugular vein, brachial plexus, thyroid, vagus nerve and many other cranial nerves are located within this region.
- The primary reasons to use cups here are to stimulate lymph drainage and to *gently* address muscles of the anterior neck, such as the sternocleidomastoid, scalenes, platysma and others.

Axilla Region

Use *only* very light suction (if any) with the lift-and-release technique in the axilla region (the armpit). This area should not be worked too aggressively due to its thinner tissue and superficially exposed vascular and lymphatic structures.

- The axillary nerve, brachial plexus and many lymph nodes are located within this region.
- The primary reason to use cups here is to stimulate lymph drainage.

Antecubital Region

Use *only* very light suction with the lift-and-release technique in the antecubital region (the front of the elbow). Cupping done in this area should be minimal due to its thinner tissue and superficially exposed vascular and lymphatic structures.

- The brachial vein, brachial artery, median nerve, median vein and lymph nodes are located within this region.
- The primary reason to use cups here is to stimulate lymph drainage. Use caution when addressing elbow issues.

Femoral Triangle

Use lighter suction in the femoral triangle, which is a small space adjacent to the groin area. Any work in this area shouldn't be too strong or aggressive due to superficially exposed vascular and lymphatic structures. Also, working in this area can seem invasive or personally uncomfortable.

- The femoral artery, great saphenous vein, femoral nerve and many lymph nodes are located within this region.

- The primary reasons to use cups here are to stimulate lymphatic drainage or to *gently* address the musculature located in the upper leg (for example, adductors, quadriceps, hip flexors). Be mindful of working too intimately in this region; working within the femoral triangle may cross the giver and receiver's comfort zone and feel too personal or potentially violating. If unsure, it's recommended not to use cups here.

Linea Alba

Use *only* light to medium suction in the linea alba, a band of tissue that connects the muscles of the abdomen and runs down the midline of the front of the body.

- The abdominal and descending aortas are located within this region, as well as the xiphoid process (lower sternum).
- The primary reasons to use cups here are to stimulate lymph movement, address the colon (especially the transverse colon section), or address the abdominal muscles.

Popliteal Fossa

Little to no cupping should be performed in the popliteal fossa (the knee pit). If any cupping is done in this area, use *only* the lightest suction to stimulate drainage of fluids. Make no attempts to manipulate other tissue structures here (the anterior cruciate ligament, or ACL, meniscus, etc.).

- The popliteal artery, peroneal nerve, tibial nerve and lymph nodes are located within this region.
- The primary reason to use cups here is to stimulate lymphatic drainage.

Kidneys

Cupping should be minimal directly over the kidneys. Suction that is too strong can be dangerous to their attachments and potentially cause fluids, such as blood, to be drawn out of these vital organs. The adrenal glands, located directly above the kidneys, could also be irritated, potentially affecting their release of chemicals (for example, aldosterone, cortisol, adrenaline). While the musculature directly over the kidneys responds well to cups, strong suction should be avoided and stationary placements should not be made for more than 2 to 3 minutes.

Temporal Region

Do not use strong suction or stationary cups in the temporal area. While cups may be used to address the temporal muscle, such applications are possible only in the area toward the hairline and to the side of the outer corner of the eye. Be sure to work with extremely detailed attention to the anatomy of this region.

- The temporal artery and some facial nerves are located within this region.
- The primary reason to use cups here is for decongestion (movement of fluid), and applications should be light. If the temporal artery is protruding, do not allow cups to slide over this area at all — skip over this area with the cup.

EVALUATION: CENTER ON THE PERSON, NOT THE CONDITION

Cupping is a therapeutic tool that can be adjusted in many ways to treat various conditions. From stress relief and muscular pain to more complicated, pathological conditions like fibromyalgia (read later in this chapter about working with fibromyalgia), cups can be helpful in countless ways. What's most important when treating with cups is that during treatment you evaluate the person as a whole and not just the medically defined condition. There are no universal protocols with therapeutic cupping.

Self-Care Applications

The best way to judge your suitability for this type of bodywork is either to check with your doctor, if you are under one's care, or to go through the criteria listed earlier in this chapter to ensure that your own health fits with the suggested criteria (for example, checking to see that no medications you may be taking contraindicate bodywork. See the sections on contraindications and safety earlier in the chapter for more details on evaluating your eligibility).

Protocols When Using Therapeutic Cupping
Soft Tissue Evaluations

Treating various conditions that involve soft tissue injuries may share some common guidelines. At all times, however, it's best to assess the person individually before every treatment.

Here are a few examples of soft tissue injuries and how they should be assessed.

WHIPLASH

Is there inflammation? How sensitive is the tissue? Are there any contraindications?

If there is a lot of inflammation and pain, only light cupping is recommended — the lift-and-release technique or the lightest moving cups to initiate lymphatic drainage and reduce the superficial pain patterns. Don't apply strong cupping if the tissue is compromised.

CARPAL TUNNEL SYNDROME

Where is the pain felt? Is the pain all over the arm or just in the hand? Is there swelling in the arm?

If the pain is felt down the outside of the arm, around the elbow and into the palm and there is light swelling, treat lymphatic drainage first, then possibly use stationary cups over any pain epicenters.

STRAINED QUADRICEPS IN AN ATHLETE

Is there superficial tenderness? Is it a first-, second- or third-degree strain? Can the area be manipulated without too much discomfort?

If it is a **mild strain** (first-degree, a pain similar to overdoing it at the gym) and the person responds comfortably to hand manipulation, then cupping will work well. Gently use the cups to work the injured muscle(s), helping to wring out stagnant blood, lymph and metabolic waste (such as lactic acid) that may be lingering in tissue, thus promoting the natural process of healing.

If it's a **severe strain** (second- to third-degree tissue damage or total loss of function), then no cupping should be used. The pull of cupping could further damage the tissue, which needs to repair itself with the body's natural inflammatory response (see "Working with Inflammation" in Chapter 10 for more information).

Pathology Evaluations

Before attempting to use cupping on people who may be experiencing a medical condition, such as diabetes, Parkinson's disease or fibromyalgia, determine what you are trying to address with cupping. Since cupping cannot eliminate these medical conditions, think of cupping as an adjunctive therapy that can offer some relief and symptomatic improvement and determine which symptomatic concerns you will work to address.

EXAMPLE: FIBROMYALGIA

Fibromyalgia, which means "muscle fiber pain," is defined as unidentified pain all over the body. A person with fibromyalgia can be very sensitive to pressure, but this complicated disease varies from person to person — some people diagnosed with fibromyalgia can feel its symptoms in certain areas of the body only, such as the shoulders, others may have restless leg syndrome, while still others may suffer from mild, recurring inflammation in the areas in which they feel pain.

Some studies have indicated that fibromyalgia patients have a higher concentration of nerve endings around the capillaries in the skin than other people, which can become easily irritated if surface tensions are altered (by various pressures applied on the skin), which would explain their heightened sensitivities. Even the slightest pressure could trigger them to fire distress signals to the brain. (See "Integumentary System," page 35 for more information.)

In my experience, it is best to ask the person how fibromyalgia affects them. Are they sensitive to light touch and find it difficult to receive bodywork (and therefore light and minimal cupping), or do they respond well to deep pressure (and therefore stronger cupping is an option)? Ultimately, cupping applications should vary according to the person's sensitivity to touch and pressure.

DID YOU KNOW?

Individuals experience far too many pathologies to be able to define every one. Some lesser-known pathologies simply need to be defined, their symptoms assessed and, if needed, inquiries made to the individual's medical care professional to determine whether they can receive bodywork and, if yes, what limitations this person may have.

CHAPTER 6

Proper Equipment

TYPES OF CUPS

Many types of cups are used in therapeutic cupping. Clinicians the world over use the most popular sets, described in this chapter, in cupping therapy. Just the same, it's important to work with the kinds of cups that best suit your personal needs, preferences and budget. Some cups, such as silicone cups, for example, may be easier to apply in self-care treatments, while others, such as the manual pump sets, may have more benefits when applying them to other people because they make it easier to vary suction pressure and come in multiple sizes.

Like any other product, cups vary in quality, functionality and durability, so consumer awareness is key. Some cups are higher in quality (varying grades of plastics are more or less durable) or are made from different materials for clinical use (glass instead of plastic so the cups can be sterilized). If you are using cups for self-care purposes *only,* then your needs will not be the same as those required in a clinical environment. Every person will gravitate toward their own set of cups, just as they do when they buy an item of clothing.

Of the many types of cups and cupping devices out there, the following are most recommended. They are all simple to use, easy to clean and able to sustain the rigor of daily therapeutic bodywork. And while cups are sold in many places — health supply stores, pharmacies, bodywork educational companies and even online — it is best to purchase units from a reputable source (see Resources, page 250, for suggestions).

Safety Point

Beyond the general usage and cleaning instructions detailed in this chapter, be sure to check package information for each set of cups for their proper care.

The most popular cupping sets are the following:

1. **Manual Vacuum Pump Gun Cupping Set:** Featuring manual polycarbonate plastic cups with a vacuum pump gun, these sets are great for both professional and personal use. An easy-to-use hand-pump gun creates the desired suction and a wide variety of sizes that vary from large to very small to allow full body applications for anyone interested in receiving cupping.
2. **Silicone cups (clear or slightly tinted):** These sets are good for personal and professional use but have a small range of sizes for full body applications.
3. **Glass vacuum cups:** Due to their fragility and cleaning requirements, these sets are best for professionals.
4. **Face cupping sets:** Best for facial applications, but also for very small body parts (for example, hands) and children.
5. **Glass fire cups and vacuum therapy machines:** Recommended for professionally trained practitioners only.

If you are working on yourself, you can apply cups while standing (excluding colon work, where it is best to lie down so the abdominal muscles can relax), seated or lying down. There are also a couple of things you may want to note when using cups:

If you're working on yourself with silicone cups in the shower, be sure to apply soap to serve as the lubricant (see box, at right), but be careful not to make the floor slippery.

When you're applying cups to another person, it is best for that person to be lying down (on their back or abdomen, depending on what part of the body is being cupped) and fully relaxed to receive the treatment (see Chapter 7: "Using Cups in Treatment" for more information on how to apply them).

Proper Removal of Cup

Removing a cup should be done with just as much care as you used to apply it. Do not pull or yank the cup off the body, since this is uncomfortable (and oftentimes painful!) for the recipient. Rather, break the seal of the cup where it meets the skin by slipping your finger under the lip of the cup. With the manual vacuum pump cup sets, simply toggle the valve at the top of the cup to release the suction and then remove it. With the silicone cups, simply squeeze the cup again to remove it.

Also, be sure to remove the cup so it opens *away from the body* if you are applying it to someone else. You do not want to aim whatever may be released from cupping (toxicity, negative mental or spiritual energy, etc.) toward yourself, so that it isn't absorbed by your own body. This is an important element to grasp with cupping therapy.

❶ Manual Vacuum Pump Gun Cupping Set

(KHANGZHU BRAND, SEE RESOURCES, PAGE 250).

This generally affordable system includes:

- Polycarbonate plastic cups
- Suction pump gun
- Optional connector hose
- Connecting rubber tip(s)

The system requires moderate hand strength to use the pump gun, which creates and regulates the suction on this set. Those who use this set may find the pump gun is stronger than they anticipated. For this reason, it is recommended to flutter-pump — that is, using small, slow half pumps — to gradually increase the suction pressure as needed.

When preparing to use these cups, choose the appropriate size, lightly make contact with the skin, and pump the handle of the pump gun to create the desired suction.

PROS: Variable sizes; control of suction; good for self-care applications; cups are usually made of durable plastic material. Excellent for stationary work or multiple cup applications.

CONS: The solid, inflexible edge of these cups may prove difficult or uncomfortable when working over joints or bony landmarks. The connecting green tip, where cups attach at the end of the hose or gun, can shift out of place or stretch if it is not cleaned with soap and water when cups are being used with oil, which leads to cups slipping out of the connector easily, especially when one moving cup is attached to the hose. To prevent this, try not to rest your fingers against the connecting tip while moving cups. Instead, grip the cup around the base where it meets the skin. When cleaning, do not immerse guns or tubes in water, as they will corrode and break.

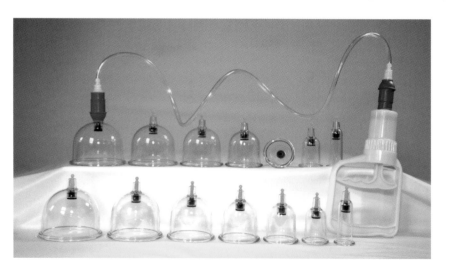

❷ Silicone Cups

Sets include squeezable silicone cups and are very simple to use. The suction is created by squeezing these pliable cups with one or both hands, which removes the air from inside the cup and creates a vacuum. Once the cup is placed against the skin, simply release the squeeze and the cup is attached. To remove the cup, simply squeeze the cup again or break the seal with your finger where the cup meets the skin — do not pull or yank the cup off, as this is uncomfortable for the recipient.

These cups come in all kinds of pretty colors; however, the clear silicone cups are preferred so you can see what's happening to the tissue while the cup is on the body. The silicone will render even the clearest of these cups slightly opaque, but you will be able to monitor changes in the tissue color through clear silicone better than through a blue or green silicone cup. The way these cups fit into your hands can also differ (a more claw-like grip with the clear ones, a more rounded grip with the orange-tinted cups), so personal comfort and preference is something to take into consideration.

One great benefit with these cups — and in contrast to the solid, full-circle edge of a plastic or glass cup — is the ability to squeeze them into somewhat distorted shapes to fit into awkward spaces. Most silicone cups can be squeezed into a more oval shape, which allows them to be placed on sometimes more challenging areas that aren't perfectly round or flat, like along the shin and ankle or over joints like the knee, elbow or shoulder.

While they seem to have a maximum suction, beware of the largest cups. These cups may have a much stronger maximum suction (the more you squeeze, the stronger the suction), so be mindful when applying these anywhere on the body.

PROS: Easy to use; pliable material allows them to be squeezed into variable forms (for example, around the ankle or along the shin); soft edges are often more pleasant around joints and bony prominences.

CONS: The largest cup can easily provide a suction that is too strong.

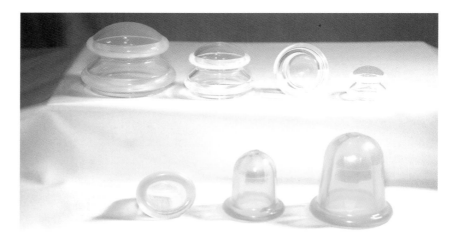

❸ Glass Vacuum Cups

Glass vacuum cups are relatively easy to use, but their composition makes them more delicate. A vacuum is created by squeezing the rubber or plastic bulb connected to the top of the cup to remove the air, then placing the cup against the skin before releasing the squeeze to create a suction on the body.

These cups have a relatively mild maximum strength suction, considering that only so much air can be squeezed out of the bulb, which prevents too much pressure from being used. And while some of the cups may feel nicer against the skin as they glide than the plastic cups do, the glass cups are breakable. Different sets also have squeeze bulbs of different colors (red is shown here) and are made of different materials, so some squeeze bulbs dry out and crack easily.

While cleaning can be a bit tedious, these glass cups are excellent and best suited for use in professional settings.

PROS: Easy to work with a somewhat constant suction; easier to grip around base of cup because of its indented edge.

CONS: Glass is breakable; not suggested for stationary cups in case they fall off. Exercise caution when cleaning (see cleaning instructions later in chapter for more information).

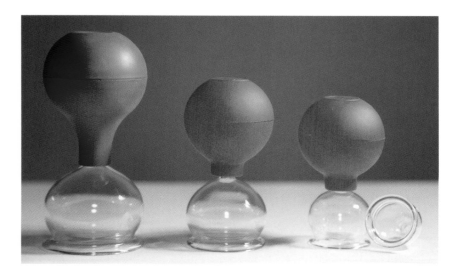

❹ Face Cupping Sets

Made of glass, these small cupping sets have a gentle and fairly moderate maximum suction because of a small squeeze bulb, so it is not likely to mark the face. Because of the heightened sensitivity of facial tissue, however, and even though this set allows for a regulated, lighter suction, if the suction seems too strong for the person, be sure to use less or use only the lift-and-release method of application (see application suggestions in Chapters 8 and 9). While these cups are most recommended for use on the face, they may also be used on small body parts, such as extremities, and on children.

To apply cups, simply squeeze the air out of the bulb, gently make contact with the cup on the skin, then release the squeeze of the bulb to create the suction. For more detailed instruction on how to use these cups, see Chapter 7: "Using Cups in Treatment."

This set requires a similar cleaning regimen to the glass vacuum cups. To the best of your ability, do not get water up inside the bulb (see "Cleaning and Storage" on page 105). Beyond the general cleaning instructions listed below, be sure to follow the cleaning instructions for each set.

There are some face cupping sets that use plastic cups. While they will work, they are not recommended. Plastic face cups break easily, cannot be sterilized to most clinical standards and can feel scratchy on the skin. They may be a more affordable option for those seeking self-care, though.

PROS: Even at maximum strength of suction on the face, there is a low likelihood of marking the face; small cups can be used on the face or small body parts (feet, hands, etc.); great for working on children, too.

CONS: Caution with cleaning. The squeeze bulbs are the area of most concern for cleaning these cups; be sure not to get water inside the bulb.

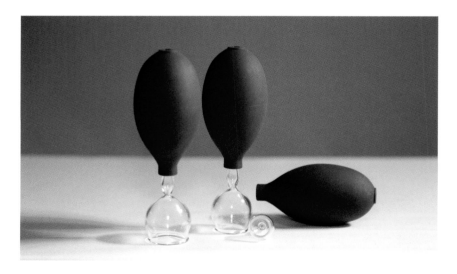

❺ Glass Fire Cups and Vacuum Therapy Machines

Both these types of equipment are less commonly used but still deserve some discussion.

Glass fire cups are among the most primitive, and that makes them attractive to some. While they may be preferred for their presumed authenticity, fire cups require a great deal of control with an unpredictable element — fire. Fire cupping is predominantly reserved for professional use by acupuncturists and Traditional Chinese Medicine practitioners, so any massage or therapeutic bodyworker choosing to use them may be working out of their legal scope of practice, which is predominantly illegal and not recommended.

Fire cups also require the confidence and dexterity to work smoothly with flaming materials and a cup, which can prove too complicated for most. They can pose another danger as well: the person applying a cup might nervously slam the cup down on a body while holding the fire's source in the other hand, resulting in pain to the treatment's recipient.

Safety Point

Fire cupping should only be used by trained professionals.

Vacuum therapy machines are excellent for professionally trained bodyworkers. These systems provide optimal control of suction pressure, from the slightest to very strong pressure, as well as some automated lift-and-release or vibration options, all of which allow for entirely different therapeutic, clinical and diversified applications of vacuum therapy. These machines can be very expensive but are well worth the investment if you use vacuum therapies regularly in a professional practice.

These units can be very harmful if used incorrectly, however — and there is a high probability for misuse with inexperience. A strong suction, for example, can easily bruise and/or cause a lot of damage to various body tissues.

All things considered, this system is *not* recommended for non-professional bodyworkers. I have purchased machines from people who have not been professionally trained yet bought them thinking that more is better in terms of suction and that, if their bodyworker worked miracles, then this device could be for them. It's a dangerous premise. To ensure proper, safe applications, those who *do* purchase these machines should receive legitimate, hands-on training before attempting to use it on anyone.

Overview of Cupping Sets

TYPE	METHOD OF SUCTION	CONTROL OF SUCTION	RELEASE OF SUCTION	CUP SIZES	EASE OF SELF-APPLICATION
Manual vacuum pump gun and plastic cups	Manual. Hand pump gun (with optional hose attachment).	Great. Hand pumping allows slight suction increase with control. Replicating desired suction is relatively easy.	Either release valves at top of cup or break the seal with a finger where the skin meets the cup.	Many sizes are available in different cupping sets.	Good. While it's relatively easy to use the optional hose for one cup work on your own body, it is limiting with certain body parts (your hands and arms). Also, a person can easily harm themselves if using too much suction.
Silicone, clear or slightly tinted cups	Manual. Squeeze the cup to create the suction.	Good. The lighter you squeeze, the lighter the suction. It can be difficult, however, to replicate consistency of suction.	Simply squeeze the cup or break the seal with a finger where the skin meets the cup.	Good variety in each set. The clear set typically has four sizes, while the orange-tinted cups have three sizes.	Great. Can be used easily and suction controlled comfortably. Can be used with oil or in the shower using soap.
Glass vacuum cups	Manual. Squeeze bulb to remove air, place cup against skin, then release the squeezed bulb to create the suction.	Good. A hand controls how strong the suction is, but getting light to medium pressure can be difficult to control and replicate.	Simply squeeze the bulb again to release.	Varied; shown on p. 100 are 2 cm (0.78 in), 3 cm (1.18 in), 4 cm (1.57 in) and 5 cm (1.97 in) wide cups.	Fair. One-handed squeeze bulb is easy to use, but glass means they break if you drop one. Recommended more for professional use.
Face (glass) cupping sets	Manual. Squeeze bulb to remove air, place cup against skin, then release the squeezed bulb to create the suction.	Great. Light, regulated suction for delicate face tissue.	Simply squeeze the bulb again to release.	Sizes and number of cups vary, generally three or four very small cups per set.	Good. Easy to use, but be careful not to drop and break the glass cups.

WHAT TO USE WITH CUPS

Lubricant

When using cups, there must be some medium between each cup and the skin to create a seal, and applied products can do just that. Cups also require a lubricant to move on the skin. A light, smooth oil (such as fractionated — non-solidifying, professional grade — coconut, sesame or jojoba) is best for sliding and ease of application. For home care, olive or avocado oil out of the pantry also works well.

Cream or Lotion

These products work well on body hair, as well as on thicker foot or hand tissue. Note that even when these products are used, cups may not adhere on thicker, callused feet or skin with excessive body hair.

Amount to Use

No matter the experience of the person applying cups, cupping requires a substantial amount of lubricant for best use, especially when attempting to slide the cups on the body. If there is too little lubricant, the cups will not move easily, and this can be painful to the person receiving the work.

How much is required? Enough to create a thin layer on the surface of the skin but not so much that the oil is dripping off the body. Apply a decent amount of oil at first, wipe it off your hands with a cloth or towel, then pick up the cups. It is easier to wipe off excess oil than to continually add small amounts. Simply apply liberally at the beginning of a treatment, as this ensures an optimal application.

Products to Use After Treatment

Therapeutic cupping increases overall circulation as well as providing relief to sore muscles, so an application of your favorite product afterwards will penetrate *deeper* into the tissue. How? Considering how cups can really "open up" body tissues by increasing vasodilation, any products you apply will be drawn into the body as circulation recedes. Topical cellulite products (such as those sold by day spas for cellulite reduction) are beneficial if that is your focus, or any pain-relieving liniment, such as arnica (a commonly used homeopathic remedy) for sore muscles, will work wonderfully. Cooling cryotherapy products, however, may be a little too cool for some people, as they can penetrate more deeply into the body. Use your best judgment in choosing a product when the temperature is cooler.

CLEANING AND STORAGE

Cleaning Supplies

All cups can be cleaned with antibacterial or antimicrobial dish soap and then air-dried. If further cleaning and sterilizing is desired — or required by regulation in professional environments — be sure to use a product that is suitable to the material the cups are made of. Rubbing alcohol, for example, works for most cups, but a stronger disinfectant (for therapy clinics, hospitals, etc.) could be corrosive to any non-glass cups. If using these stronger products, be sure to dilute them accordingly.

Specialized Cleaning

MANUAL PUMP GUNS

Manual pump guns should *not* be washed in water, because the metal coil springs inside them can easily rust. To clean a pump gun, simply wipe it down with a slightly damp, soapy cloth or approved disinfecting wipes. The hoses that sometimes come with these sets should not be immersed in water either, since any water that enters the hose will be drawn into the chamber with the springs. Wipe the hose in the same way as you would the pump gun.

SQUEEZE BULB CUPS

Squeeze bulb cups should be cleaned with caution. When washing the squeeze bulb, be sure to just *wash the outside* of the bulb and to not get water *inside the bulb.* Any water inside the bulb may cause mold to grow over time. If water does get inside the bulb, simply drip-air-dry, rinse the inside with alcohol and allow to drip-air-dry again. Try washing them with the opening of the bulb tipped down and out of the running water, and be sure to also air-dry with the opening tipped down.

Storage

In an office, it is recommended to store cups either on shelves, so they are available at the ready, or on storage carts (with or without drawers). Wheeled storage carts that can be moved easily and conveniently to the treatment area may be the best option. Any glass cups should be stored with safety in mind so they don't fall and break.

Home storage can include many options, from closet shelves to vanity cabinets. Be sure to keep a few silicone cups in the shower, for example, and allow them to air-dry when not in use — do not allow water to remain inside the cup to prevent any potential mold growth. See page 99 for more information on using silicone cups in the shower for self-care.

> ### DID YOU KNOW?
>
> Disinfecting wipes should be used only when working at an out-of-office location off-site; otherwise, they will corrode and break down any non-glass cups. Plus, they do not fully clean the cups, which can lead to cross-contamination when used in consecutive, varying body treatments. If using disinfecting wipes for on-site work (for example, at a sporting event, outside of the clinical setting), be sure to wash cups thoroughly in soap and water at the end of the day.

CHAPTER 7

Using Cups in Treatment

APPLICATIONS OF CUPS

A variety of techniques are used in therapeutic applications. From stationary cup placements to moving cups to the versatile lift-and-release technique, applications can vary tremendously depending on the area being treated, the condition being treated and the person receiving the treatment. Certain cupping techniques, however, are used for specific reasons. For example:

- Stationary cups are used to focus on a specific location.
- Moving cups work to address general areas.
- Lift-and-release cupping is used to gently introduce cups to the body and/or when other cupping methods may be uncomfortable.

When deciding on which technique to use, consider why you are offering a cupping treatment and the expected outcome. For example, are you addressing deeper, tight skeletal muscles (using a stationary cup) or are you targeting cellulite (moving cup)? Perhaps stationary or moving cups are uncomfortable for an individual, in which case you may need to use the lift-and-release technique.

As with any type of therapy, practicing technique is necessary and can only improve the results. With any of these applications, it is important to practice both the technique and the amount of pressure being used. Every person will respond differently to cupping, so be willing to adjust and learn as you practice. One person may respond wonderfully to the deeper penetration of stationary cups for sciatica, for example, while another may prefer the more stimulating sensation of light moving cups over the same gluteal region. Be sure that you have enough lubricant to move a cup smoothly, that pressure is comfortable and that the cupping experience feels good.

CUPPING 101

Practice cupping on your own body to help you better understand the differences in applying pressure on the skin. Pay particular attention to the sensation of too much (painful) pressure and adjusting accordingly so you can make adjustments when working on someone else.

Safety Point

Leaving cups on the body for more than 3 minutes is not recommended. This type of treatment is often practiced in Traditional Chinese Medicine and other alternative medicine applications, but it requires specialized training in these disciplines.

TECHNIQUES IN CUPPING

Stationary Cups

Placing — and leaving — a cup on the skin with applied suction is considered a stationary cup. Stationary cups address the exact location of their application and can be used to focus on the deeper layers of tissue. Such an application encourages slow separation of the many layers of tissue, in which cups create a lift of tissue from negative pressure, promote blood vessels to dilate and slowly pull fluids toward the skin's surface. This process allows tissue fluids to slowly seep into the spaces being created between layers of tissue, hydrating from the inside out and perhaps releasing anything stagnant, such as old blood, as the area softens. Stationary cups can be used to slowly dredge what may be embedded within these layers of soft tissue and bring deep, replenishing hydration into the area. For detailed instructions on how to attach cups to various areas of the body, see Chapter 8: "Basic Applications for Common Conditions."

The length of time that a cup remains on the body or the strength of applied pressure can yield different results, too. Those new to using cups should begin by applying them for shorter amounts of time and with lighter pressure, whether it is the first experience with cupping or the initial application to a specific body part. Allow the tissue to become acclimated, perhaps 30 seconds to a minute at first. In subsequent treatments, cups can be applied to the body for 2 to 3 minutes at a time, in many cases, to yield greater results.

SUCTION PRESSURES WITH STATIONARY CUPS

How much pressure, or suction, is used depends on the purpose of the treatment and the comfort level of the person receiving cups. It ranges from light to strong suction.

Think of stationary cups as decompressing and separating tissues while stimulating the movement of fluids exactly where they are applied. Short durations are optimal here, as putting the cups on for an excessive amount of time — 5 to 10 minutes — can create stagnation and perhaps even trauma. Instead, remove them after they've been applied for a few minutes, allow the body to process and assimilate the changes that have occurred, and then consider reapplying them after evaluating the skin and the person. Remember, cups are meant to encourage circulatory movement within the body, not concentrate or block it.

DID YOU KNOW?

Cups can have an effect as much as 4 inches (10 cm) into the human anatomy. Stationary cups create a deeper sense of penetration over the specific location on which they are applied, perhaps accompanied by stronger suction.

Moving Cups

Moving cups are exactly as they sound — cups that are attached to the skin and moved over the surface of the body. Moving cups work to address the more superficial layers, down to muscular tissue and even some visceral organ applications, such as when addressing the colon. Moving cups are more about the lift and manipulation of the cup in your hand, and less about the strength of suction — there is no need to use stronger suction to address deeper anatomy because the tension created by lifting the cup as you move it is intended to reach into deeper layers of tissue. Moving a cup offers a new dimension of treatment and sensation that varies from a stationary cup. Sliding cups along the body's surface creates a wave-like effect, making a significant difference within the tissues.

The Benefits of Lifting a Cup on the Body

Whenever a cup is attached to the body, adding a little lift of tension creates a sort of reflective reaction *into* the body, meaning that a slight lifted tension can affect the more superficial tissues with lighter suction pressure, while a somewhat higher lifted tension with the same lighter suction pressure can reach deeper into the muscles and visceral organs. Rather than using strong suction to access the deeper layers, lift the cup to bring about such results.

Suction Pressures with Moving Cups

Apply only light to medium suction pressure when moving the cup; otherwise, you can damage the tissues. Be sure to lift the cup as you move it; do not press it into the body. Once adhered, lift the cup until you feel a slight tension and then slide it along. While pushing the cup along the body offers some relief, the greatest benefit comes with the enhanced lift and stretch of the cup as you move it along. This is easy to feel, both by the one receiving the sensation as well as the person applying the cup.

You should never feel any "ripping" or "tearing" as you move the cup. If you or the recipient feel anything like this, stop using the movement.

CUPPING 101

A moving cup should slide with ease and be comfortable to the recipient. If this is not possible, consider using the lift-and-release technique to facilitate moving a cup. Also consider using this technique over any "speed bumps" while trying to move the cup smoothly along any line of movement. Never force a moving cup; rather, address restricted tissue obstacles as needed.

Consider using lighter suction to move the cup or the lift-and-release technique to facilitate any desired movements.

How Do You Use This Technique?

- Attach the cup to the skin using light to medium pressure; the more sensitive the person, the lighter the suction should be.
- Gently lift the cup away from the body until you feel a slight tension engage.
- While maintaining this hold, slowly begin to slide the cup across the surface of the body.
- Then release the tension and release the cup from the body.
- Do not just yank the cup off — it will hurt.

Here are some additional guidelines for optimal cup movement:

- Apply oil or approved creams liberally to the body to allow the cups to move with ease and without discomfort (for example, tugging the skin). Using more product on the skin so there is enough lubricant to slide the cups comfortably typically works better.
- If the cup still sticks onto the skin while moving it, even after following these instructions, you have likely discovered a restriction under the surface. Once you have identified this "speed bump" in an area otherwise moving fluidly, address this newfound obstruction by using other techniques discussed in this chapter, such as lift-and-release, a stationary cup or skilled hands, like a massage therapist, along with some alternatives explored in this book.
- Initial applications can be somewhat sensitive for a multitude of reasons, including dehydration, scar tissue, adhesions and others, so move the cups carefully. Everyone is very different, so if cupping hurts, be sure to respect that reaction. The mentality here is not "no pain, no gain." While the feeling of cups is pretty much indescribable, it should be a welcome experience for the body.

How Fast Do You Move the Cups?

The speed at which you move the cups can cause different reactions, too.

1. *Moving cups slowly can be soothing and sedating.*
This style is good for long draining strokes, relaxing applications, slow separation of tight tissue and as an initial application to allow the body to acclimate to this sensation.

2. *Moving cups at a faster pace can be stimulating.*
This speed can be used to really energize tissue or break up areas of congestion, such as cellulite. Faster paces are generally more sensitive and can easily border on painful, so be sure to use lighter suction the faster you go.

Slower paces and variations on *how* the cups are moved (the twist of a cup along the IT band, shaking a cup over the belly of a muscle as you slide the cup along its length, or the lift of a cup to mimic a cross-fiber friction for scar applications) can offer a truly unique experience with modern cupping therapies.

> ### THERAPEUTIC THOUGHT: MASSAGE MOVEMENTS
> *I liken moving cups to massage therapy — slower movements are relaxing and can be used for deeper applications, while faster movements are more stimulating and are used to treat more superficial tissues.*

Lift-and-Release

When stationary cups are too intense, lift-and-release can quickly encourage a gentle lift, separation and hydration of the tissues that may be too sensitive or irritated at first. Working the surface tissue in this manner can gradually and positively affect all the tissues in the region and pave the way for eventually welcoming the stationary cup.

This technique is a powerful adaptation of both stationary *and* moving cups, but it is a more gentle and fluid movement. You are literally "pumping" the tissue with a cup to facilitate quick changes in hydration, tension and pliability. Think of lift-and-release as milking the tissue into a healthier state.

It can be a beneficial application all on its own or be used to make stationary or moving cups more comfortable and effective.

DID YOU KNOW?

The Morse Code of Cups, a method of communication that uses a series of dots and dashes, can be seen as an analogy for cupping. The Morse code combines sliding movements (dashes) with the quick-fix lift-and-release (dots) techniques.

- On its own, it can be used to treat an entire area of hypersensitivity (for example, fibromyalgia), or lymphatic drainage can be easily mimicked when following correct drainage pathways (see Chapter 9: "Therapeutic Cupping for Lymphatic Drainage" for more information).
- When used with moving cups, it can address a tight "speed bump" along the way to promote overall softening of tissue that may be too restricted, compromised or sensitive. I often refer to this as the Morse Code of Cups due to the combination of slides and sudden lift-and-releases.
- When a stationary cup is too intense during an initial application, this technique can provide an alternative to a stationary cup.
- When you want to see more immediate, positive responses in the body, lift-and-release cupping can offer a good, gentle option.

How Do You Use This Technique?

- Attach the cup to the skin.
- Apply light to medium pressure; the more sensitive the person, the lighter the pressure should be.
- Gently lift the cup away from the body until you feel a slight tension engage.
- Maintain this hold for a minimum of 1 second to a maximum of 10 seconds.
- Then release the tension and release the cup.

Repeat these steps a few times in the same location to milk the tissue or apply to an entire area for an overall, regional effect. The more sensitive or compromised the tissue is, the more delicate the cupping should be. Lift-and-release enables the person to respond to cups more quickly and comfortably.

Flash Cupping

This technique involves repeatedly applying multiple cups (minimum 2, maximum 6) over an area of the body without leaving them in place for long. While the cup may remain on the tissue like a stationary cup, the timespan it is left in place should be much shorter. It's also different from the lift-and-release technique because it uses multiple cups in a quicker succession of applications. This technique is used most often with pulmonary applications over the back (due to the way it stimulates the mucociliary escalator of the lungs from this location) but can easily be altered to treat other parts of the body, for example the shoulders and IT band. (See "Pulmonary Conditions and Cupping" on page 238 for step-by-step application of flash cupping.)

WHEN TO USE LIGHT, MEDIUM OR STRONG SUCTION

It's a common question: How much suction pressure should I use? There is no one answer. As with other types of bodywork and applicable therapies, there are many reasons to use different pressures. And every person you work on will respond differently to each pressure applied.

For example, why is it that a well-defined bodybuilder who asks for very deep tissue massage can have barely any suction applied without discomfort, while a woman in her 90s can have medium strength pressure applied with moving cups and experience comfort and pleasure. There could be countless reasons why — hydration, inflammation, and elasticity of the tissue are some. Once again, this question is best answered with your own approach; however, here are some common suggestions on how to assess suction pressure.

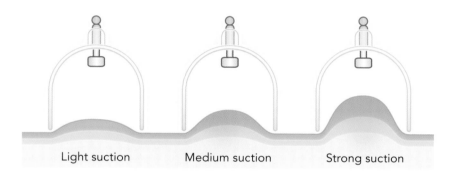

Light suction   Medium suction   Strong suction

THERAPEUTIC THOUGHT: PEG THE PRESSURE

Think of pressures as being applied in the same way as in massage therapy: the deeper the pressure, the slower the movements, if any. If a massage therapist is using an elbow to address deep muscles in the hip, for example, the application is very specific. The deeper the pressure, the less movement, if any.

Light Suction

SUPERFICIAL LYMPHATIC DRAINAGE

True superficial lymphatic drainage causes no hyperemia (redness) in tissue, and this is difficult to accomplish with anything but a professional-grade cupping machine. For this reason, follow the *intermediate* lymph drainage pathways in Chapter 9 (see page 201) as guidance.

✪ TECHNIQUES TO USE: Lift-and-release, moving.

VERY SENSITIVE TO THE TOUCH

If clients are in a great deal of pain, extremely sensitive to the touch or have an underlying pathology that causes hypersensitivity, such as fibromyalgia, very light work can have some benefits. Start with the lift-and-release technique to introduce the suction, and apply stationary or moving cups only when the person is calm, relaxed and receptive to this light suction. Be sure to ask how the suction pressure feels throughout the application.

✪ TECHNIQUES TO USE: Lift-and-release, moving or stationary. If using stationary placement, be sure to check in about pressure.

ACUTE INFLAMMATION

Any initial application of cups around compromised tissue (for example, post-surgical inflammation) should be light and with the intention of encouraging the movement of lymph fluids.

✪ TECHNIQUES TO USE: Lift-and-release, moving. Remember, acutely inflamed tissue should not be directly cupped.

EMOTIONAL TRAUMA

With so many possible contributing factors (traumatic experiences, loss of a loved one, depression), working with your hands and cups can provide one of the most soothing and therapeutic experiences, and lighter work can yield some remarkable results.

✪ TECHNIQUES TO USE: Lift-and-release, moving (slowly) or stationary.

Medium Suction

DEEPER LYMPHATIC DRAINAGE

If you are working to dissolve cellulite or chronic edema or support sports recovery — and the person is comfortable with the stronger-than-lighter suction — then medium pressure is a good option. Consider the multiple functions of cups moving along drainage pathways, dissolving and liquefying stagnant areas within the superficial fluid-moving layers, bringing materials that may be embedded in tissue to the surface *and* encouraging lymph movement for disposal. This movement of cups should be smooth and not painful to the recipient.

✪ TECHNIQUES TO USE: Lift-and-release, moving.

RIGID, THICKER TISSUE

Anytime tissue feels thick, restricted or rigid, you may choose to begin with medium suction. Whether an individual is a construction worker, an office clerk or your average body generally in good health, the texture of one's tissues will vary considerably from person to person.

The upper back and shoulders, for example, can often carry a lot of tension and have a thicker texture on some people. Therefore, be sure to take into consideration each individual and their lifestyle and habits (hydration, exercise, nutrition, smoking, sun exposure, etc.), which may contribute to the thicker tissue. The dermis is thicker on the back of the body than on the front of it. The dermis is thickest on the bottom of the feet and hands and thinnest over the eyes.

While it is usually suggested to try light suction first, thicker tissue may pose a challenge. The lift-and-release technique can be used to encourage an overall loosening of the area. Stationary cups will help with slow, constant drawing of blood (and lymph) into the area. Medium-suctioned sliding of the cups will feel like good deep massage movements across any area you work.

✪ TECHNIQUES TO USE: Lift-and-release, moving or stationary.

Safety Point
....

Blood and lymph respond simultaneously to applied cups. Thicker, more dehydrated tissue may welcome the increased fluid exchange and rush of blood into the area, but be sure not to leave cups on for too long so you don't *create* stagnation of lymph.

CHRONIC INFLAMMATION

Medium suction is beneficial when trying to draw inflammation out of an area (not flared up inflammation). Stationary cups around a chronically inflamed joint (such as the knee) can draw out the inflammatory agents, followed by a comfortable suction to move the cups in the proper direction for drainage (for example, the knee up to the groin and into the lower inguinal lymph nodes). (See Chapter 9 for more detailed information on how to approach this subject.)

✪ TECHNIQUES TO USE: Stationary (for drawing chronic inflammation out of an area, such as knee joint), lift-and-release. The moving cup that removes inflammation from any area should be lighter suction pressure.

MASSAGE, THERAPY AND BODYWORK MOVES

Any applied moving techniques should be less about the suction and more about the lift of the cup to affect the underlying tissue. While many people think that deep tissue bodywork (and a little pain) is one of the only ways to achieve resolution of many soft-tissue restrictions (like tight muscles), this is not the case with cups. *Again, cups should never hurt.* While cups can yield some rather impressive results on their own, consider them an adjunctive, complementary tool to the work you do. For example, I can use one or two cups with ease to mimic kneading through the shoulders and upper back with a comfortable medium suction, and all the while the recipient feels a great depth of pressure within their body.

Consider manipulating the tissues *through* the cup.

✪ TECHNIQUES TO USE: Lift-and-release, moving or stationary.

THERAPEUTIC THOUGHT: CREATIVE APPLICATIONS

For bodyworkers, once you become comfortable using cups, mimic massage techniques to add variety to treatments. Just as the hands can work across muscle fibers with frictions or knead tight muscles, a similar application with cups can add benefits to these areas. Be creative with how you choose to use the cups, keeping safety in mind as the priority. I personally like the feeling of a smaller cup moving with slow friction across tight shoulder muscles, just as fingertips would. Often, people cannot distinguish between the two.

Strong Suction

PRIMARILY FOR STATIONARY CUP APPLICATIONS ONLY

Strong suction should be applied only after you have introduced a lighter suction. Initial applications using strong suction can absolutely cause traumatic damage to tissue. If cups have been repeatedly used, however, such as on regular clients who receive cupping with every session, immediate application of stronger pressure in subsequent sessions should be fine.

REGULARLY MANIPULATED MUSCLE TISSUE

For those people who are accustomed to therapeutic bodywork, starting with strong suction may be fine. While it is always suggested to build up to strong suction pressure, there will be people who respond well to immediate strong suction, such as athletes who receive regular manual therapies.

THICKER, CALLUSED TISSUE

The thicker tissue on feet or hands often poses a difficulty with almost any suction, but deep suction can bypass the dermal challenges here and get into the deeper layers more quickly and with greater ease.

✪ TECHNIQUES TO USE: Lift-and-release or stationary.

Keep in mind that after any strong suction applications, it is highly recommended to do some circulation-encouraging movements (whether with hands or lighter cups).

USING CUPS AS A MASSAGE AND BODYWORK TOOL

In the field of massage and bodywork, countless applications of cupping can be added to enhance a therapist's scope of work. What influences the addition of cupping is the practitioner's intention, along with their knowledge and skillset of techniques and uses. Here are some things to consider when assessing the inclusion of cups to complement existing bodywork therapies:

- Do you find a tense area that could benefit from enhancing superficial circulation and overall loosening? Addressing stress or tight muscles, for example, can benefit from moving cups.
- Are you looking to focus on certain areas with friction or petrissage-like (kneading) techniques? When addressing trigger points ('knots' in muscles), for example, a stationary cup with a constant tension lift will allow you to move the cup (not slide it) in small circular or cross-fiber friction-like movements.
- Is there fluid retention you want to drain from an area? To assist lymphatic drainage, gentle, rhythmic and repetitive movements of lift-and-release or moving cups in the proper direction of drainage can be helpful. (See Chapter 9 for more information on proper lymphatic drainage directions.)
- Is there an area that could benefit from slow, soft tissue decompression? Stationary cups can offer relief by not pressing further into an already compressed environment, such as in the case of sciatica.
- Or are you working on an area that could benefit from a soothing, even distribution of nourishing blood flow *after* work has been done, such as lightly using cups to soften an entire area after tender trigger points have been addressed?

Cupping with Other Therapies

Therapeutic cupping is considered a manual therapy and therefore can be employed by any licensed professional who practices therapeutic bodywork, but it is important to work within one's scope of practice, too. For example, an esthetician should use cups only for more superficial circulation and lymphatic drainage but not attempt to apply cups in a massage therapy-like manner.

Chances are, if you're working on a patient or client with your hands, cups can safely be added with beneficial results. For physical therapists, massage therapists and personal trainers, cups can be an adjunctive therapy that brings a new element of relief and release to treatments. Cups can help enhance same-session (results within one session) results, too.

MASSAGE THERAPIST

Cups can greatly enhance massage therapists' treatments. Cupping allows therapists to conserve their often over-exerted efforts by more quickly creating warm, pliable tissue, especially if their client has thick skin, dehydrated tissues, large muscles, etc. Therapists will be able to see and feel the change in their client's tissue. Cups can bring a new sense of therapeutic potential that may not have been possible without exerting effort or with other therapeutic techniques.

PHYSICAL THERAPISTS

Physical therapists may have treatment protocols that require their patient's tissue to be warm and pliable before attempting any rehabilitative exercises. This alone can take time, but cups can accelerate this process. The client is then ready for exercises with less effort exerted by both the patient and therapist.

SPORTS TRAINERS

Sports trainers aim to keep their athletes in peak performance condition, and cupping is an effective adjunct to achieve this. From clearing lactic acid overload to repetitive motion restrictions, cups may keep athletes going and their muscles in a state of optimal functioning, both before and after an event.

Multi-Tasking

Using cups at the same time as applying another bodywork therapy is another alternative. If a patient shows a lot of tension in one shoulder, for example, cups could be set in place on that shoulder while the therapist works elsewhere on the upper back. Keep in mind the amount of time that cups are left on the body and monitor the cups as you work.

THERAPEUTIC THOUGHT: FEEL THE TISSUE

*Regardless of how cups are incorporated into a clinician's body of work, I always encourage them to feel the tissue with their hands and assess the area first before placing cups, then again after applying cups. They'll be able to feel if the tissue is warmer, softer or looser and apply their professional training to work this area further if needed. However, I also caution therapists **NOT to overwork the client**. Ambition can sometimes override logic when you see how quickly change can occur. Remember that most compromised tissue didn't just happen overnight, so respect the cumulative process in all bodywork.*

Insight for Bodyworkers

Cupping might also reveal what the hands might not feel or confirm what has already been suspected. Here are some examples of how cups can offer further insight to therapists:

- As they are locating the more restricted musculature around a compromised joint, cups may mark the tissue with different colors and potentially lead to further discoveries.
- Cups may show unseen or buried areas of dysfunction. Various colors, textures, temperatures and adhesions might be seen on the skin after cupping and reveal what is happening under the surface, which may not be seen with non-invasive therapeutic treatments.
- Markings from cupping may provide photographic documentation. If the person being cupped is working with an insurance company, for example, the effects of cupping could be documented after a series of treatments to chart progress. If the person is simply curious about the effects of cupping, photographs of marks or adhesions can offer more insight about the state of their condition.

EMOTIONAL RELEASE WITH CUPS

Emotions in the Physical Body

Emotional stressors are known to contribute to physical, mental and emotional disorders. Many faculties (medical institutions, universities, alternative health practices) have shown that emotional traumas can be stored within the various cellular structures of the body (organs, skin, muscles, endocrine glands, tissue, etc.), only to be accessed and potentially released when said cellular structures are manipulated by various methods of therapeutic bodywork. Pharmacologist Candace Pert (www.candacepert.com), for example, did extensive research into how the body stores emotions at the ends of neuropeptide receptors within the soft tissues of the body; epicenters of these neuropeptide receptors within the body are called nodal points.

While the limbic system is the center for processing emotions in the brain, emotional traumas may become imprinted in various cells of the body — as deeply as DNA — where some traumas have occurred. Whether it be a physical (for example, a car accident) or emotional trauma (such as an abusive relationship), the body and mind stimulate the fight-or-flight response at the time of the incident. When this occurs, all the body's relevant hormones, such as adrenaline and cortisol, are released into the system and the body races to take care of the stressor.

Anatomy FYI

Peptides are organic compounds that are formed by certain combinations of *amino acids*. The body contains 16 amino acids, and in various organizational patterns, amino acids make up virtually every structure of the body.

Neuropeptides are chains of amino acids that are created from nerve cells within the brain. An example is endorphin, which the body produces in response to pain.

Neuropeptide receptors are the specialized cells that receive these neuropeptides at a different point of necessity in the body. With endorphins, if there is an area of pain, the body produces endorphins and sends them to the receptors in the necessary location.

The process is similar to how hormones are produced and delivered to designated locations in the body.

When trauma settles, there is still the emotional memory of the experience, now imprinted within various soft tissues of the body because it could not be processed naturally at that time. The inability to process this material may form a sort of storage within the body systems to contain it. Osteopath Dr. John E. Upledger (www.upledger.com) refers to this type of phenomena as a somato-emotional cyst or energy cyst.

The body prioritizes survival skills, and the locations where these emotions were embedded into one's anatomy may retain this traumatic information until it is released, either by bodywork, breathing exercises or other possible therapeutic releases. Left untreated, such manifestations may eventually lead to a multitude of physical dysfunctions — structural imbalances, exhaustion, chronic pain patterns, inflammation responses — or even altered immune system functions. The medical field has established a specialized study of this phenomenon called psychoneuroimmunology.

Storage in Connective Tissue

Therapeutic release of these emotional traumas can be accessed by manipulating connective tissue. This extremely strong, permeable and conductive material is woven into every structure of the body and can store energy associated with emotional trauma. When therapeutically manipulated, connective tissue can provide a point of access to wherever such materials may be hiding. Renowned physical therapist John F. Barnes, (www.myofascialrelease.com) founder of myofascial release therapy, for example, has demonstrated this therapy helps to release the memories of trauma from somewhere in the connective tissue network with dramatic therapeutic results, such as crying and recalling the traumatic event.

Working with Emotional Releases

Cupping has some rather dynamic potential for therapeutic releases of all kinds, and this emotional aspect should also be considered. Whether intended or not, there is the potential for emotional releases — as with most bodywork — and one should be prepared. While many emotional entities can be "held in," "suppressed" or "buried" in the body, the cups have the capability to potentially release this material and bring it to the surface.

Consider this information when working with cups: Always be aware of how the recipient is responding to the work. Does their breathing change? Do they become disoriented? Do they suddenly begin to move away from the work? Is there a sudden urge to cry? While these releases can be very therapeutic and beneficial, a therapist must sympathize with the person's reaction to this aspect of the healing process and work accordingly.

Safety Point

Strong, vigorous cupping is absolutely *not* recommended when there is an emotional release happening during the treatment.

Significance of Cups Reactions

- **Marking behind the left shoulder, behind the heart:** Often the coloring can be a pink or light red speckling, signifying a more recent emotional distress (sudden loss, a recent stressful moment in the person's life, etc.), or a darker coloring, signifying an older containment of emotions that is being released.

- **Outpouring of emotions:** Cups can open the proverbial Pandora's box of emotional releases, so be aware and supportive should this occur. This is a welcome therapeutic occurrence and is necessary for healing if this is the case with a client. People may cry, become disconnected or disoriented and become extra sensitive physically during such times, so be sure that suction pressure is adjusted accordingly.

- **If using the cups for self-care, be mindful of how you are feeling within your own body.** Any similar reactions you may be experiencing are welcome. If this becomes an overwhelming process, however, be sure to seek help from someone, either a professional or a friend or loved one, to talk with about your feelings.

- **Energy levels:** Emotional distress naturally has a draining effect on the energy levels of the entire body system. Consider this when using cups on people with low energy, as cups tend to lower the body's overall energy. Be mindful that they will be able to leave the session with enough energy to perform their normal daily activities.

PART 3

TREATING COMMON CONDITIONS WITH CUPPING

CHAPTER 8

Basic Applications for Common Conditions: Therapist and Self-Care Options

OVERVIEW OF THERAPEUTIC CUPPING

DID YOU KNOW?

Considering individual sensitivities, one person may require strong stationary cup applications to get relief, while another person may reap more benefit from a lighter, more overall moving cup application for the same condition. There is no *one cup fits all application*.

Therapeutic cupping is one of the most versatile methods of bodywork. When used in various applications and techniques, cupping can offer supports for the body's systems. It can stimulate circulation, support tissue hydration, clear areas of congestion and help the body rebuild healthy tissue, among other supports. Cupping can also be modified to suit the needs of many individuals afflicted with a host of conditions, with treatments that range from the lightest lymphatic drainage treatment to deeper muscular maneuvers.

A variety of cupping equipment and applications are used to treat certain conditions. Some applications offer a host of benefits to specific conditions, but some techniques may be adjusted.

In treating neck and shoulder tension, for example, some individuals are more responsive to deeper manipulation — like deep tissue massage therapy — at first (applied stationary cups along the upper shoulders to release some neck tension), some individuals prefer that the surface tissue be warmed up before attempting to work deeper (gentle moving cups over the shoulders and posterior neck region), and still others respond better to an even lighter application (the lift-and-release technique across the entire region).

WHAT YOU NEED TO KNOW

The applications demonstrated in this chapter are tried-and-true treatments that have benefited corresponding conditions. Applications for each condition are marked as:

- **Primary applications:** the most common applications of cupping.
- **Optional applications:** alternative treatments to the common, primary applications. When treating carpal tunnel syndrome, for example, a number of locations can be causing discomfort, therefore, a range of available applications are offered as suitable treatments.

Body Positioning

Each application will include instructions regarding the suitable position of the body for applying the cups, whether to someone else or used in a self-care treatment. The two most common positions are:

- **Prone**, or lying face down.
  The easiest way to apply cups to the lower back is when the person is in the *prone* position.

- **Supine**, or lying face up.
  The easiest way to apply cups to the abdomen is when the person is in the *supine* position.

If applicable, other positions will be suggested for some applications, for example, the side-lying position for the self-care treatment of sciatica.

Regions of the Body

When working on different body parts, certain terms are used to better define the intended location or instruct a person applying cups to somebody else.

The following terms are used in the step-by-step instructions for cup applications:

Proximal means *closer to* a certain point, or *closer* to the torso.
- The upper arm is more *proximal* to the torso than the lower arm.
- The knee is more *proximal* to the torso than the ankle.

Distal means *further from* a certain point, or *further from* the torso.
- The wrist is more *distal* than the elbow.
- The lower leg is more *distal* to the torso than the upper thigh.

These terms are used regularly when cupping the limbs, especially when addressing lymphatic drainage or when locating certain points on the body.

Lateral means more to the outside or away from the midline of the body.
- *Lateral* epicondylitis is pain felt on the outside of the elbow joint.
- The IT band is on the *lateral* part of the thigh.

Medial means more to the inside or closer to the midline of the body.
- *Medial* epicondylitis is pain felt on the inside of the elbow joint.
- The adductors are on the *medial* part of the thigh.

Anterior refers to the front of the body.
- The endangerment site in the front of the neck is called the *anterior* triangle.
- The *anterior* superior iliac spine (ASIS) is where your fingertips typically rest when the hands are placed on the hips, the high hip points in the front of the pelvis.

Posterior refers to the back of the body.
- The popliteal fossa is an endangerment site in the *posterior* aspect of the knee.
- The *posterior* iliac crest is the area where you will locate the high points on the back of the pelvis, where your thumbs may reach when the hands are on the hips.

CHOOSING THE RIGHT CUP

With so many cups available, it can be difficult to decide what type of cup to use and where to use it on the body.

The question I'm often asked is, *"Which cup should I use for ____?"* And my answer is typically, *"It doesn't necessarily matter which cup you use, but how you use it."* While certain cups are better than others for some applications — such as silicone cups in the shower, glass squeeze ball cups in professional settings, face cups for detailed face work — it matters more that you are comfortable using the cups you have. One person may like the grip of a silicone cup in their hands and how easy it is to apply by simply squeezing it, while another may prefer the manual vacuum pump gun for its ability to create various suction pressures and its greater variety of cup sizes. While this book will demonstrate applications using two sets of cups (a manual pump gun with plastic cups and silicone cups), any cups can be used similarly to accomplish these applications.

Manual vacuum pump gun cups are best used for:

- **Most stationary cup placements:** This system offers the convenience of multiple cup sizes. The cups, which are typically made from clear polycarbonate plastic, allow greater visibility of surface tissue reaction, both when placing them on the body and during the time they are attached.
- **Some self-care applications:** The optional hose allows for some variability in certain areas (e.g., the back of the neck).
- **Some lift-and-release optional applications:** The gun's suction control is helpful in certain areas (e.g., the front of the neck, or anterior triangle).

Silicone cups best used for:

- **Most self-care applications:** These cups are easy to use for quick applications and home use.
- **Most moving cup applications:** Their comfortable grip is a benefit when moving cups. Manual pump gun cups can also move, but they take some getting used to (such as not resting the finger against the connector bit and overall comfort in the hand).
- **Some stationary cup applications:** Silicone cups are more comfortable around joints (e.g., the knee joint), near bones or where stationary placements may be more challenging with a manual pump gun (e.g., the palm of the hand, base of the foot).
- **Some lift-and-release applications:** The smaller silicone cups are ideal for more delicate regions (e.g., the anterior forearm, for carpal tunnel syndrome).

Mixing and matching cupping sets is also an option.

What Size Cup Should You Use?

When choosing the size of a cup, be sure to pick one that fits the area of the body being treated (larger or smaller body parts), as well as the intention of the application (specific or more general applications).

LARGER CUPS

Large cups are best for initial applications and larger muscle areas, such as the back, shoulders and abdomen. The size of these cups allows you to first address regional surface tissue and warm up the area before working on focused applications. Just like in massage, where you would start a treatment with the palm of your hand before using your thumb, in cupping you would work on a larger area before focusing on a particular point. If you begin with a small cup on a larger area, such as the gluteal region, it is not only extra sensitive, but the initial, focused suction could also cause tissue damage. Using a larger cup also allows you to see what is happening to the tissue more clearly while the cup is attached. Are there visible adhesions? Is the tissue changing colors? Assessing tissue changes tends to be more challenging when using smaller cups.

SMALLER CUPS

Small cups are best for focused work and smaller body parts. While a large cup cannot be used on smaller parts of the body, such as the neck, arms and feet, there are various sizes of cups in between, so choose a size that best fits the area you are working on. Once a general area has been warmed up, focusing the application with smaller cups enables a more detailed effect; for example, cross-fiber friction into rhomboid muscles or trigger point isolations.

Before You Begin

Be sure to have a lubricant of choice (fragrance-free oil or cream) ready to apply before attaching any cups. Lubricant helps create an optimal seal when attaching the cup to the skin, and an ample amount of lubricant is necessary when attempting to move any cup across the skin's surface.

For more information on stationary versus moving cups, as well as treatment positions, techniques and suction pressure, see Chapter 7: "Using Cups in Treatment," page 106.

HOW TO APPLY AND REMOVE CUPS

Knowing how to properly apply and remove cups is essential to maximize healing and minimize potential injury. The equipment used to demonstrate applications here, either plastic cups with a manual pump gun or clear silicone cups, is proven safe and effective for all cupping applications demonstrated. If you are using other therapeutic cups for these applications, be sure to receive proper training on how to apply and remove them safely.

Applying Plastic Cups with a Manual Pump Gun

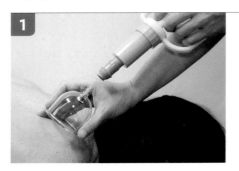

1 With the pump gun in one hand and desired size of cup for the area being treated in the other, approach the area of application.

Note

The top of the cup has a valve (yellow here).

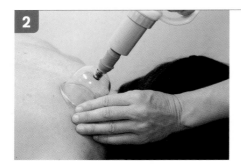

2 Place the connector piece (green here) directly over the valve at the top of the cup, in direct contact with the skin. There is no need to press the cup into the body; simply make contact with the surface.

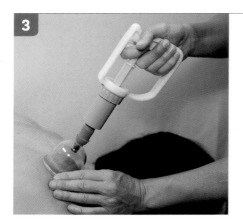

3 Pull the handle up to create the suction. The pump gun removes air from the cup through the valve at the top of the cup. This action closes the valve, allowing the gun to be removed and leaving the cup in place with suction established. The more you pump the gun's handle, the stronger the suction will be.

Note

If you pull the handle and no suction occurs, remove the gun and manually release the valve (shown in yellow) to open it; you may hear an audible "click" as it releases to the open position. Valves may be closed on new cups or after cleaning. The pump gun cannot remove air to create suction if the valve is already closed.

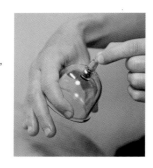

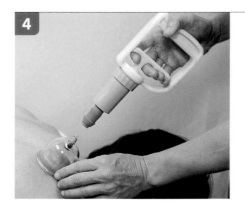

4 Remove the gun by lifting it straight off the cup. Do not bend the connector to the side when removing the gun. Making contact at the top of the valve as you attempt to remove it may release its seal, thereby releasing the suction.

Removing Plastic Cups with a Manual Pump Gun

Be sure not to yank or pop the cup off — this can be unsettling to the body, as well as annoying to the person receiving the treatment.

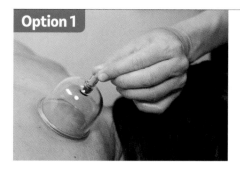

Option 1

Release the valve at the top of the cup to break the seal. Lift the cup and remove.

Note

Remember to open the cup away from you. Whatever may have been released — for example, negative energies or pathogens — should be directed away from your own body when applying cups to someone else so you do not personally absorb any of it.

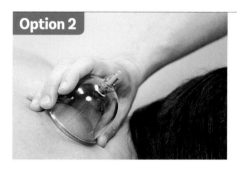

Option 2

Slide a finger under the lip of the cup where it meets the skin to release the seal; the ring finger (fourth finger) is used in this example.

Note

Be sure that a fingernail does not dig into the skin while doing this — it will hurt.

Applying Plastic Cups with a Manual Pump Gun for Self-Care

While it may be possible to apply cups to your own body with only the pump gun, most cupping sets will have an optional attachment hose. If so, this is useful for self-care applications.

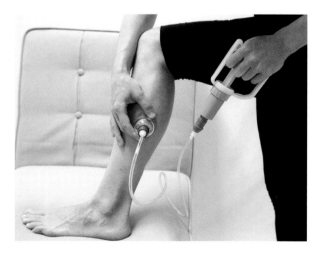

Applying Silicone Cups

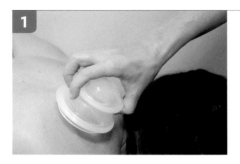

1 Choose the desired size of cup for the area being treated.

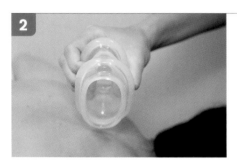

2 Squeeze the cup to remove air. The more you squeeze, the stronger the suction will be.

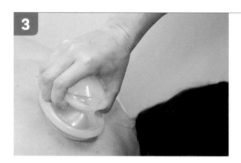

3 Keeping the cup squeezed, place it against the skin.

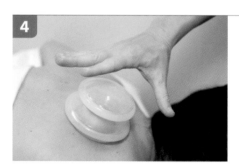

4 Release the squeeze. The cup is now adhered to the skin.

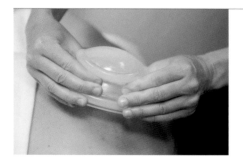

TWO-HANDED SQUEEZE OPTION: Grip the cup on either side using two hands. Squeeze the cup with both hands for application and removal.

Removing Silicone Cups

Be sure not to yank or pop the cup off — this can be unsettling to the body, as well as annoying to the person receiving the treatment.

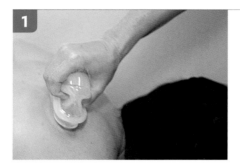

Simply squeeze the cup to release the suction.

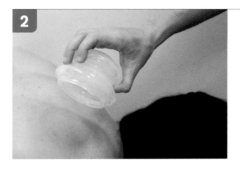

The cup is now removed.

Applying Silicone Cups for Self-Care

To apply and remove silicone cups in self-care applications, follow the instructions above.

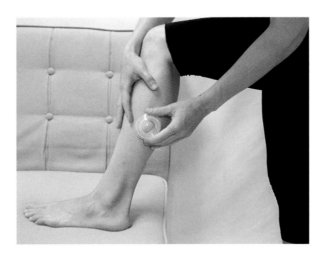

LIMITATIONS IN USING CUPS

Surface Tissue and the Lymphatic System

Some people may have more challenged surface tissues and lymphatic systems that cause hypersensitivities to initial cupping applications. Dehydrated tissues, trapped inflammation, solidified lymph, toxic histories (such as addictions) or overstimulated nerve endings are just a few of the reasons why deeper applications may not be comfortably received.

If you are attempting to use cups on a certain area — to relieve sciatica, for example — and you have checked for all contraindications and applied the lightest of stationary cups but the person is still uncomfortable, consider working just the surface this first time with either moving or lift-and-release techniques to see what may change in the individual's comfort. When working with the lymphatic system, treating just the surface tissue will help affect change within the deeper levels of lymph vessels, as well as all other deeper tissues like muscles, as they are all interconnected. (See Chapter 9: "Therapeutic Cupping for Lymphatic Drainage" for more information on addressing the lymphatic system.)

Cups could create more congestion or stagnation with the lymphatic system if you ignore someone's hypersensitivity and force any cupping applications. Addressing these surface tissues first whenever someone is initially hypersensitive will provide greater results with any (later) cupping applications.

Safety Point

Cups are all about creating fluidity within the tissue layers of the body. Do not apply full strength on an area to get maximum benefit if the body simply isn't welcoming the application of cups. Some of the most rewarding cupping experiences have come from the lightest of applications.

TREATING COMMON CONDITIONS WITH CUPS

BACK, NECK AND SHOULDER APPLICATIONS

The aches and pains felt in the back, neck and shoulders are among the most common physical discomforts. With so many causes contributing to tension in this area, it is one of the most notable regions of the body for receiving various therapies and medical attention, from massage therapy to physical therapy and chiropractic care to pain medications and various surgeries.

Therapeutic cupping not only offers fantastic results on its own but also complements other forms of therapeutic bodywork. In this section, applications are targeted to deal with stress relief and overall back tension, neck and shoulder tension, and lower back pain. Adjustments to address associated discomforts will be made where possible.

Safety and Contraindications

One of the primary contraindications for working in this area is compromised vertebrae; more specifically, bulging, herniated or degenerative discs. While many people don't have an ideal spinal posture, be sure to ask the recipient if they know of any vertebral issues that have been diagnosed or any specific locations that are painful to touch. Also, use your own visual assessment before considering the application of cups; for example, take note of and use caution with any visual deviations in the spinal column the recipient may not be aware of. Do not use cups on any of these potentially compromised vertebral structures.

Evaluate the Spine

A basic, quick and helpful way to evaluate the spine is by palpating with your fingers. By gently walking your fingers down the spinous processes, as well as alongside the spine, one vertebra at a time, you can identify any areas that may be compromised or overly tender and should be avoided. This process by no means replaces proper medical diagnosis, but if any location is painful to the touch, cups should not be applied directly over that specific location. Instead, consider applying cups around the area if desired.

Stress Relief and Overall Back Tension

Ask how stress manifests itself in the body and most people will point to back, neck and shoulder tension. This tension potentially has a deeper effect on the central nervous system, too, and therefore impacts the entire body.

Causes

Stress can be caused by physical, mental or emotional situations. Regardless of how stress manifests itself in the body, millions of people have used massage and similar bodywork to help alleviate it.

Symptoms

Individual symptoms of stress can be as unique as a snowflake. There may be physical discomforts, such as sore or tired muscles and headaches, as well as exhaustion and depression. Many people "carry their stress" in their back, neck and shoulders.

Cupping and Stress Relief

The back is a common area to work with cups for relief. Cups should be applied in a soothing manner. Think of cups as being disorienting to tight areas stuck in a state of contraction, and the naturally decompressive sensation of cups can be a welcome relief. Once cupping begins to take effect, the peripheral repercussions can have profound effects on the entire central nervous system. People have described cup applications as creating more "breathing room within their bodies."

Cupping and Overall Back Tension

To address overall back tension where stress is not a major factor, the same applications can be used. However, suction may be stronger for stationary cups, and the pace may be slightly faster for moving cups.

Techniques

LIFT-AND-RELEASE APPLICATIONS can be applied slowly down each side of the spine and repeated as often as you like, for a maximum of 10 and a minimum of 2 minutes.

MOVING CUPS in the same region with lighter pressure can be very soothing, and the softening tissue can be easily palpated.

STATIONARY CUPS can be positioned along the sides of the spine, using lighter suction for stress relief, or stronger suction for more intense muscular applications.

Conditions that may also benefit from these applications:

- Postural imbalances (e.g., scoliosis)
- Some cases of fibromyalgia
- Tension headaches
- Compressed, entrapped or pinched nerves
- Parkinson's disease
- Multiple sclerosis (not during active flare-ups)
- Cerebral palsy

Note

All applications for the back will be in the prone position.

Primary Application

ALONG THE SIDES OF THE SPINE (STATIONARY CUPS, PRONE POSITION)

TARGET AREA INCLUDES: Portions of the upper, middle and lower trapezius, rhomboids, erector spinae, paraspinals, latissimus dorsi, serratus anterior and quadratus lumborum (QL) muscles, as well as the aponeurosis along the spine and all peripheral nerves that pass through this region.

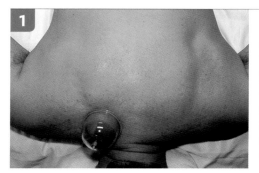

Place the first cup to the side of the spine, between the upper shoulder blade and the upper thoracic vertebrae area. To locate the starting point, lightly touch the spine at the base of the neck with your fingertips and walk the fingers over to the top corner of the shoulder blade on whichever side you chose to begin the application. The soft tissue space in between those two bony locations is where you should place the first cup. Do not place the cup directly on the spine or the shoulder blade.

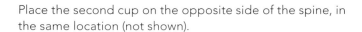

Place the second cup on the opposite side of the spine, in the same location (not shown).

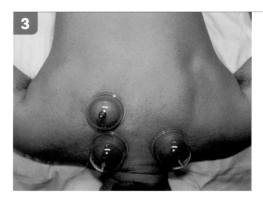

Place the next cup directly below the first cup along the side of the spine.

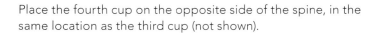

Place the fourth cup on the opposite side of the spine, in the same location as the third cup (not shown).

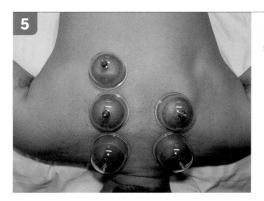

Place the next cup directly below the third cup along the side of the spine.

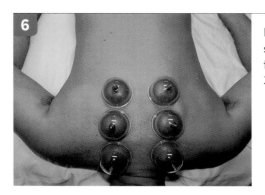

6 Place the sixth cup on the opposite side of the spine, in the same location as the fifth cup. Allow cups to remain in place for a maximum of 3 minutes but no less than a minimum of 30 seconds.

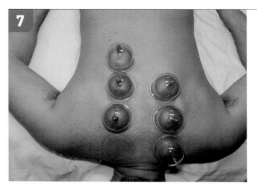

7 Using the cup first applied (#1), remove it and place cup #1 below the last bottom cup, on the same side of the spine (cup #5).

Think of "walking the cups" down the back to get this application moving. Release each cup in the order in which it was placed, and then reapply it in the same order as you place them further down the spine.

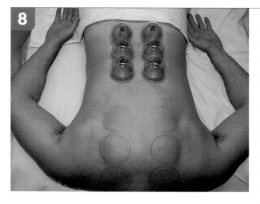

8 Continue "walking the cups" down the back, removing cups sequentially and applying them to the next location down each side of the spine, until you reach the base of the spine/ sacrum and hip bones.

The location of the two bottommost cups, at the sacroiliac (SI) joint in the lower back, is where you will stop. To locate it, place the fingers at the base of the spine where it meets the sacrum (tailbone). Lightly walk the fingers out to each side a short distance (approximately 2 fingers' width). The slight divots here are the SI joints. Cups should be placed over this area, but make sure they are not directly over the spine when attached.

SHOWN HERE: All cups replaced at the end point, just at the SI joints and posterior iliac crest (back hip bones). Allow cups to remain in place for a maximum of 3 minutes but no less than a minimum of 30 seconds. Remove cups one at a time, in the order they were applied for the best relief. The process may be repeated 2 or 3 times, if desired.

Note

Suction pressure should be light to medium over kidneys. (See "Endangerment Sites," page 92, for more information.)

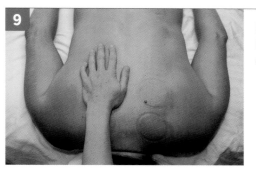

9 **RECOMMENDED AFTER STATIONARY CUPS HAVE BEEN REMOVED:** Use either your hand or a cup to lightly encourage recirculation.

Optional Application

FULL BACK TREATMENT
(MOVING CUPS, PRONE POSITION)

This application of moving cups mimics a wave-like effect — similar to massage strokes — along the length of soft tissue around the spine, or when stationary cups are not welcome. Place cups along either side of the spine. It is recommended to use light or medium suction pressure for moving cups.

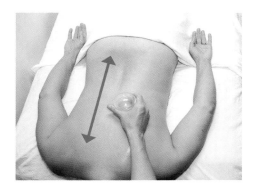

- Begin with lighter suction. As the tissue softens, you may increase the pressure if desired.
- Attach the cup lightly in between the shoulder blades on either side of the spine, then gently lift the cup away from the body until you feel a slight tension engage.
- Slowly slide the cup up and down the back along either side of the spine. The topmost point should be positioned between the top of the shoulder blade and the spine; the bottommost point should be just before the hip bones.
- This line of movement may be repeated a few times.

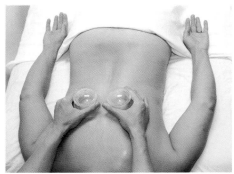

SELF-CARE APPLICATION

Self-care application isn't an option here because the anatomy can be challenging. Have a friend or loved one help you apply the cups, get a massage, do some yoga, or take a bath and relax!

Note

A moving cup may "stick" when attempting to slide over the kidney region (at the base of the rib cage on both sides alongside the spine). Do not force any moving cup. If necessary, detach the cup over this location, use the lift-and-release technique to address the sticking point — a sort of speed bump — and continue with the moving cup (like the Morse Code of Cups), or use even lighter suction pressure to move cups across this location.

Neck and Shoulder Tension

The neck and shoulders are a very common area for tension. All the muscles within this region commonly hold tension, contributing to discomforts in the neck and shoulders. It is important to properly assess causes of individual tension and apply cupping accordingly.

Causes

Causes vary widely, and individuals experience tension and pain very differently. Examples of contributing factors to neck and shoulder tension include whiplash, temporomandibular joint (TMJ) dysfunction syndrome, ergonomic challenges at work (such as computer jobs), poor posture patterns, depression, dehydration, sleeping patterns, bulging or herniated discs or generally tight muscles.

Symptoms

Pain can be dull and aching, sharp and shooting (if so, check with a medical professional for a possible pinched nerve or other structural issues), limited and/or painful range of motion, headaches or overall stiffness in the neck and shoulder region.

Cupping and Neck and Shoulder Tension

Cups can promote overall softening, pliability and decompression to otherwise tight and restricted tissues in such a small area. Tension headaches, for example, can be relieved with even minimal cupping.

One of the greatest benefits of using cups in this area is that they can alleviate symptoms without unnecessary pressing on small, tight muscles. Instead, cups can manipulate them with negative pressure to allow relief.

Techniques

LIFT-AND-RELEASE APPLICATIONS in the region of discomfort is a good introductory application, especially if a person is overly sensitive or has a lot of discomfort.

MOVING CUPS can be used over the posterior (back) side of the neck (behind the ears), down through the shoulders. Suction pressure should be light, and the pace should be slow or medium for maximum comfort and ease of movement.

STATIONARY CUPS can be placed all over this posterior (back) upper shoulder region. Stationary cups are not recommended directly on the back of the neck, as this region is too small, complex, and close to the Anterior Triangle endangerment site (see "Endangerment Sites" in Chapter 5, page 92, for more information). Also, never place any stationary cups in the front of the neck.

Conditions that may also benefit from these applications:

- Headaches
- Temporomandibular joint (TMJ) dysfunction
- Whiplash
- Torticollis (also known as 'wry neck,' chronic muscle spasms in the neck region)
- Thoracic outlet syndrome (nerve compression in the upper chest, neck and shoulder region where many nerves exit the spine and enter the arm, neck and shoulders)
- Carpal tunnel syndrome

Primary Application

NECK AND SHOULDER (STATIONARY CUPS, PRONE POSITION)

TARGET AREA INCLUDES: Portions of upper, middle and lower trapezius, rhomboids, levator scapula and supraspinatus muscles.

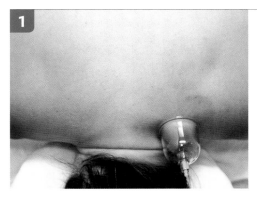

1 Place the first cup where the neck meets the shoulder. To locate the starting point, place the fingertips lightly on the spine at the base of the neck, then walk the fingers over toward the top of the shoulder blade on the side you chose to begin with. At a slight angle, place a cup at the point in the soft tissue space where the neck joins the top of the shoulder.

If you find a "knot" in the soft tissue as you feel around (this is a common area for such tension), this is the best location to place the cup.

In the proper location, the cup should not be directly over the spine or over the shoulder blade bone.

2 Place the second cup on the opposite side of the spine, in the same location (not shown).

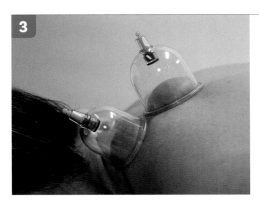

3 Place the third cup directly below the first cup, along the same side of the spine, in between the shoulder blade and spine. Note the difference in angles between the first and third cups. This cup is more on the back line of the body, rather than at the top of the shoulder where the first cup was placed.

4 Place the next cup on the opposite side of the spine, in the same location (not shown).

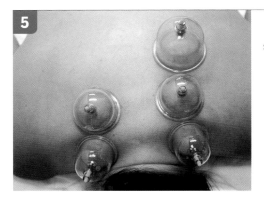

5 Place the next cup directly below the third cup, along the side of the spine.

6

Place the next cup on the opposite side of the spine, in the same location (not shown).

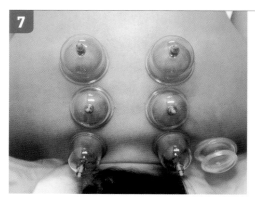

7

Place a smaller cup to the lateral side of the first cup, medial to the acromioclavicular (AC) joint, at the top of the shoulder. To locate this point, follow a straight line from the ear toward the shoulder joint, passing the first cup in place. There will be a small bump of bone, about one hand's width away from the side of the neck. This is the AC joint. Place the cup on the inside of the joint, just to the outside of the first cup applied.

Note

Different cup sets are used in the photo. While it is not necessary to own both sets, a silicone cup is more pliable and may fit better over this boney shoulder region.

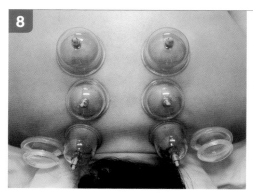

8

Place another cup on the opposite shoulder, next to the second cup, in the same location as the seventh cup. Allow cups to remain in place for a maximum of 3 minutes but no less than 30 seconds. Remove cups one at a time, in the order they were applied for the best relief.

SUGGESTED AFTER REMOVING ALL STATIONARY CUPS: Apply soothing massage strokes where cups were applied.

Optional Applications

ADDITIONAL STATIONARY CUPS

Two additional cups may be placed directly over the center of each shoulder blade.

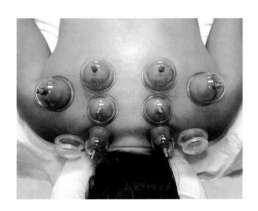

For those who have front-rounded shoulders, this application addresses very tight shoulder muscles (infraspinatus, teres minor and major). The area may be surprisingly sensitive, so be mindful when applying cups.

▸ To find these additional locations, draw a diagonal line from the armpit crease up to the first and second cups placed.

▸ Next, draw a straight line from the third and fourth cups straight out toward the armpit crease. Where these two imaginary lines intersect is the location for these cups. This location is directly over the scapula and addresses the infraspinatus muscle.

▸ If you're still having difficulty locating this point, lightly rub into tissue to feel for tight bands of muscles in this area. Where you feel the most tension over the shoulder blade is where you should place these additional cups.

ACROSS THE BACK OF NECK AND UPPER SHOULDERS (MOVING CUPS, PRONE POSITION)

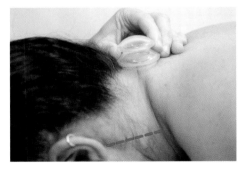

TARGET AREA INCLUDES: Upper trapezius, levator scapulae and many smaller (often tense) erector spinae and suboccipital muscles of the neck.

This application of cups is used to mimic massage-like strokes over the back of the neck and upper shoulders, and offers relief when stationary cups are not comfortable.

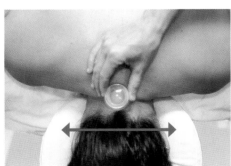

▸ Begin with a lighter suction; as the tissue softens, you may increase pressure if desired.

▸ Attach the cup lightly in the lower neck area, then gently lift it away from the neck until you feel a slight tension engage.

▸ Slowly slide the cup side to side across the back of the neck (top); progress down into shoulders if desired.

▸ This line of movement (side to side across the back of the neck) may be repeated a few times. Be sure to stay behind the ear to keep cupping out of the anterior triangle endangerment site (bottom).

▸ This can be a very tense area, so move slowly and pay attention to extra-tight areas.

FRONT OF THE NECK (SUPINE POSITION)

Using cups in the front of the neck offers great relief to this region, which may hold a lot of tension, but be aware that this is the site of the anterior triangle (a major endangerment site discussed in Chapter 5, page 92).

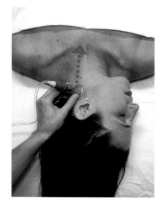

The anterior triangle — although an endangerment area — contains integral muscles (sternocleidomastoid, scalenes, platysma) that contribute to neck and shoulder tension. It often requires manipulation for optimal resolution, from tension within the temporomandibular joint (TMJ) or whiplash. This sensitive area responds very well to even the lightest suction applications where finger manipulations on such anatomy may be uncomfortable. This is meant to be very light and gentle cupping.

- Use *only* the lift-and-release technique. Absolutely no stationary or moving cups are to be used.
- Use *only* light suction — cups should be used to apply a gentle lift to tight muscles. Excess suction can cause harm to the many blood vessels and nerves that lie close to the surface here.

Example: In this case, a manual pump gun with a plastic cup is being used. The pump gun allows for more control of suction than a silicone cup. Lightly pump the handle of the gun to control gentle suction.

TARGET AREA INCLUDES: The sternocleidomastoid (SCM), scalenes and platysma muscles.

▸ Use the lift-and-release technique with only lighter suction in this region.
▸ Apply (NO SLIDING!) the cup in only this direction: down the neck, from the head toward the chest.
▸ Apply the lift-and-release on the entire front of the neck, starting up near the ear and ending down at the clavicle collarbone.

Note

Do not apply cups to any obvious vascular bodies (anything pulsing).

Safety Point

Do not use cups directly over the spine if there is any history of bulging, herniated or compromised discs.

SELF-CARE APPLICATIONS

Self-care applications may be a bit challenging, as you may be using the muscles of the upper shoulder area that attach around the neck to apply cups.

The most comfortable equipment to use may be the manual pump gun. Try to relax your arm down by your side — seated or standing — while working in the neck area.

USING A MANUAL PUMP GUN

Seated is preferred, but standing is okay, too.

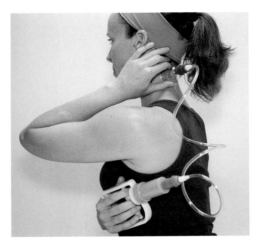

OPTION 1: Apply a cup and use the lift-and-release technique or moving cups down the back of the neck toward the shoulder.

OPTION 2: Use only the lift-and-release technique to address the front of the neck in the anterior triangle region. NO STATIONARY OR MOVING CUPS HERE.

See previously suggested applications for more detailed instruction on treating these areas.

USING SILICONE CUPS

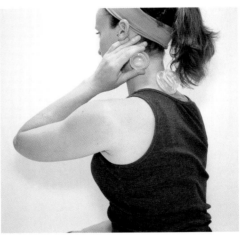

OPTION: Place a stationary cup in the tense upper shoulder area.

OPTION: Use a smaller cup to address the back of the neck and into the shoulders.

OPTION: Use a small silicone cup to address the delicate anterior triangle region with the lift-and-release technique only if desired. NO STATIONARY OR MOVING CUPS HERE.

See previously suggested applications for more detailed instructions on how to work these areas.

Low Back Pain

When we refer to back pain, it is most likely in the lower back. A lot of pressure and movement is expected from the muscles in this area, while an impressive amount of tension is placed on the bony structures that make up the lower back region.

The lower back is the support center of our bodies. At the base of the spine we find the sacrum and coccyx. The pelvis attaches to the base of the spine, and the legs that move us through daily life attach to the pelvis. Any postural imbalances, overexertion, emotional traumas or other contributing factors can lead to low back pain.

Causes

Low back pain can be caused by a multitude of contributing factors, including tight muscles, lack of flexibility, obesity, pregnancy, herniated discs or damage to muscles, ligaments and bones, to name a few. Causes for low back pain should be properly diagnosed by a health-care professional before attempting to work with cups.

Symptoms

Pain, which can be dull aching or sharp and burning, muscle spasms, sensitivity to touch in the region, difficulty standing or walking. Pain can radiate into surrounding areas or stay local. Pain that either radiates into surrounding areas or stays local are among the most common symptoms. Low back pain can be similar to sciatica pain, too.

Cupping and Low Back Pain

Cups can stimulate hydration to the soft tissue within this region, promoting softening and pliability, offering considerable relief. Cupping can also offer decompression to these weight-bearing, often fatigued anatomical structures (muscles, ligaments, bones, joints, etc.).

Techniques

THE LIFT-AND-RELEASE TECHNIQUE is a beneficial introductory application, especially if the person is overly sensitive or in a lot of pain.

MOVING CUPS can be used all over this area. Slide up and down on either side of the spine, across the entire gluteal and pelvic region, or over the sacrum and lower, lumbar spine if not contraindicated; add in a slight twisting motion if traversing over bony structures to help with the transition.

STATIONARY CUPS can be placed along lower back muscles and gluteal region.

Conditions that may also benefit from these applications:

- Postural imbalances (e.g., lordosis)
- Spinal region inflammations (e.g., ankylosing spondylitis)
- Sciatica
- Restless leg syndrome

Note

Considering the bracing and compensation that often happens within the gluteal region, placing cups here can help when addressing low back pain (see the applications for sciatica on page 164 for more options).

Primary Application

EITHER SIDE OF THE SPINE AND SACRUM (STATIONARY CUPS, PRONE POSITION)

TARGET AREA INCLUDES: Lower portions of paraspinal and transversospinalis muscles, quadratus lumborum (QL) muscle, portions of gluteus muscles, ligaments of the sacral and lumbar region (such as iliolumbar) and the sacroiliac (SI) joint.

1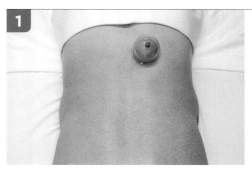
Place the first cup to the side of the spine, over the sacroiliac (SI) joint. To locate it, place the fingers at the base of the spine where it meets the sacrum (tailbone). Locating one SI joint at a time (on whichever side you chose to begin with), lightly walk the fingers out to the side a short distance, approximately 2 fingers' width, where there will be a slight divot; this is the SI joint.

Cups should be placed over this area, but make sure they are not directly over the spine when attached.

2
Place the second cup on the opposite side of the spine, in the same location (not shown).

3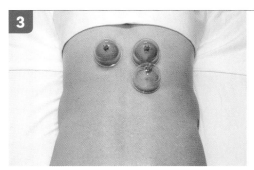
Place the third cup just above the first cup, along the same side of the spine.

4
Place the next cup on the opposite side of the spine, in the same location (not shown).

5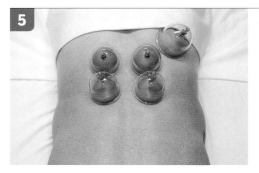
To place the fifth cup, follow a diagonal line from the first cup down toward the top of the hip joint, where you feel a bone moving when twisting the leg in and out. Place the cup diagonally next to the first cup, in the space between that cup and the hip joint. This application addresses a part of the gluteal region.

6
Place the next cup on the opposite side of the spine, in the same location (not shown).

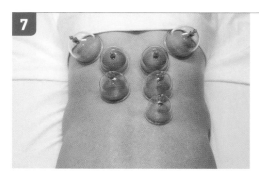

7

Place the seventh cup just above the second cup, directly over the quadratus lumborum (QL) muscle insertion and just below the 12th ("floating") rib.

The floating rib is sometimes difficult to locate; an approximate measure of its location is the length of one hand's width up from the hip bone.

Note

The suction should not be too strong here, as the kidneys are located in this area. See "Endangerment Sites," page 92, for more information.

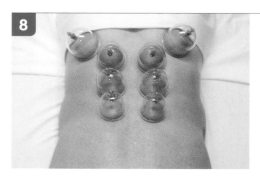

8

Place another cup on the opposite side of the spine, in the same location. Allow cups to remain in place for a maximum of 3 minutes but no less than 30 seconds. Remove cups one at a time, top to bottom, for the best relief.

SELF-CARE APPLICATION

Treating low back pain with cups on your own can be tricky and sometimes counterproductive. However, here are a few considerations:

- It may be difficult to squeeze the silicone cups behind you at such an awkward angle. The best option for using silicone cups in this region may be to lie on your side and address the gluteal region, as demonstrated in the section on sciatica on page 163. Be sure to address both sides of the spine and sacrum if attempting this application.
- The manual pump gun with its optional connector hose may be easier to use. Whichever method you try, be sure not to torque your body too much, as this can cause further discomfort. While it may prove a bit awkward, the Primary Application is possible for self-care. However, stationary cups directly to the spine and sacrum is *not* recommended for self-care due to the complexity and cautions associated with it; try a few applications and see what works for you, or ask for a friend's help.

UPPER AND LOWER EXTREMITY APPLICATIONS

These applications are targeted at the most common upper and lower extremity ailments, including frozen shoulder, elbow problems, carpal tunnel syndrome, sciatica, IT band restrictions, knee problems and plantar fasciitis. Adjustments to address other associated discomforts will be made where possible. Applications to treat IT band restrictions, for example, can be adjusted to address issues in the quadriceps, hamstrings or adductor muscles.

One of the key considerations for working on any extremity is circulation. Any stationary cups can potentially interrupt the body's natural circulation of blood and lymph, which can be potentially harmful for overall circulation. In particular, on the limbs where recirculation is naturally challenged by gravity (or other factors like a sedentary lifestyle), be sure to keep safety in mind when working to address any soft tissue restrictions with any stationary cups.

Cupping should proceed here in a centripetal direction, meaning working toward the torso. Considering the natural challenge of recirculating blood and lymph in the limbs and the significant effect cups have on moving fluid, it is important to continuously move cups toward the trunk for optimal circulation. If not, swelling could be created.

Most manual therapies, such as massage, work with the same directives for the same reasons. Gravity has enough effect on the limbs and circulation — be sure that any cupping helps and doesn't harm.

THERAPEUTIC THOUGHT: TOWARD THE TORSO

I witnessed someone who was working with carpal tunnel syndrome and repeatedly moved the cup down the forearm, from elbow to wrist. After just a few strokes, the recipient's wrist was quite swollen. I also watched someone working on their own ankle and calf, moving the cups up and down the shin and always finishing his movements down toward the ankle. Again, his ankle swelled considerably after just a minute of work.

Frozen Shoulder

Frozen shoulder, also known as adhesive capsulitis, is a condition characterized by inflammation in the lining of the joint (capsule), which leads to the formation of scar tissue in the surrounding muscles, tendons and ligaments.

Causes

Frozen shoulder can be caused by trauma, immobilization (for example, recovering from a broken arm), diabetes, poor posture or other undetermined reasons.

Symptoms

Frozen shoulder has three known stages of symptoms. In the first, painful ("freezing") stage, there is overall pain in the area and it may increase in both intensity and location, in particular at night, when lying down on the affected shoulder. During the second, stiffening ("frozen") phase, there is a more constant pain in the joint and movement is limited, which could result in the muscles beginning to waste away due to lack of use and a restricted range of motion. The third, "thawing" phase of the condition may be marked by an increase in the range of motion as the pain decreases, while there may be some recurring discomfort as the shoulder continues to thaw.

Cupping and Frozen Shoulder

Cups can be placed around the joint to draw out the embedded inflammation, increase hydration and suppleness of all soft tissues affecting the joint, and create a sense of openness or expansion in the compressed area. The range of motion may improve after cups have been applied, even more so if a therapist manipulates the joint afterwards.

Techniques

LIFT-AND-RELEASE can be used for initial applications if a person is feeling very sensitive over the affected joint when stationary cups are used. Alternatively, use this technique to initiate gentle lymphatic drainage to help clear any superficial congestion that may be causing such surface sensitivities.

MOVING CUPS can also be used to encourage lymphatic drainage, as well as to gently slide over the area if it is too sensitive for stationary cups, or with slightly stronger pressure to loosen up surrounding musculature (for example, the deltoid muscles).

STATIONARY CUPS can be placed all around the shoulder joint.

Conditions that may also benefit from these applications:

- Rotator cuff inflammation
- Bursitis
- Tendonitis, also known as tendinitis
- Thoracic outlet syndrome
- Carpal tunnel syndrome
- General shoulder joint tightness
- Tenosynovitis
- Fibromyalgia (symptomatic in the shoulder joint)

Note

Treatment can vary, from physical therapy and rehabilitation to anti-inflammatory medications and surgery. It is important to get proper medical diagnosis to ensure the condition is being treated properly.

Primary Applications

SHOULDER JOINT (STATIONARY CUPS, PRONE POSITION)

TARGET AREA INCLUDES: the shoulder joint, most rotator cuff muscles (supraspinatus, infraspinatus, teres minor and major), portions of the triceps brachii, the middle and posterior deltoid muscles and the AC joint region.

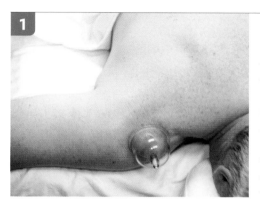

1 Place the first cup at the top of the shoulder joint, which is accessible in this position. To locate it, follow a straight line from the ear downward and out toward the arm, where you will find the top of the shoulder joint, about 3 fingers' width lateral to the acromioclavicular (AC) joint. The AC joint will be a small bump of bone where your scapula hooks onto the clavicle (collarbone) in the front.

If you are having difficulty finding this spot, lift the arm up to the side of the body. As the arm rises, there will be a small divot, or dip, at the top of the shoulder joint — this is where the first cup should be placed.

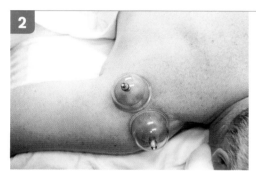

2 Place the second cup directly below the first cup toward the armpit, with the edge of the cups touching each other so the entire joint is covered.

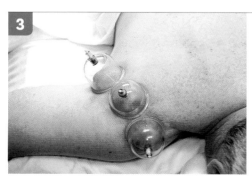

3 Place the third cup directly below the second cup and just ending where the armpit begins. Allow the cups to remain in place for a maximum of 3 minutes but no less than a minimum of 30 seconds. Remove cups one at a time, in the order they were applied for the best relief.

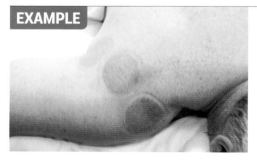

EXAMPLE In this case, the person suffers from chronic frozen shoulder. Cups remained in place for only 1 minute because the tissue turned red quickly, so this was a fast release. Quick releases of just 1 minute can be equally effective, depending on the person's condition.

The skin's redness here was warm to the touch (significantly warmer than the surrounding tissue, which typically signifies the release of inflammation).

SHOULDER JOINT (STATIONARY CUPS, SUPINE POSITION)

TARGET AREA INCLUDES: Portions of the middle and anterior deltoid, pectoralis major, biceps brachii and coracobrachialis muscles and the bicipital groove (see Anatomy FYI, below).

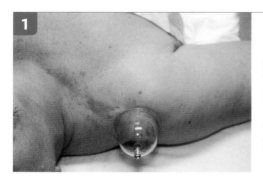

1 Place the first cup at the top of the shoulder joint, which is accessible in this position. To locate it, see Step 1 in the prone position (in the supine position, it is easier to find). The clavicle (collarbone) goes straight to the AC joint (the little bump of bone), where the first cup will be placed. Raise and lower the arm out to the side of the body to find the exact divot if necessary. This is where the first cup should be placed.

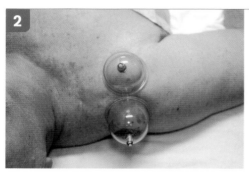

2 One cup at a time, apply cups across the entire surface of the joint that is accessible, with the edge of each cup touching so the entire joint is covered, starting at the top of the joint and working down toward the armpit.

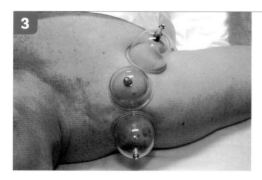

3 Allow cups to remain in place for a maximum of 3 minutes but no less than a minimum of 30 seconds. Remove cups one at a time, in the order they were applied for the best relief.

Anatomy FYI

The bicipital groove is a bony landmark on the humerus (on the upper arm) where the pectoralis major, teres major and latissimus dorsi muscles attach. The biceps brachii, coracobrachialis and anterior deltoid muscles pass through this region, as do the brachial plexus and major arteries and veins of the upper extremities.

While this region holds a lot of tension, cupping in this area should not be too strong or aggressive to avoid causing damage to the blood vessels and nerves contained within this region.

SELF-CARE APPLICATION

In a seated position, place silicone cups over the entire shoulder joint. Here, silicone cups are typically used because they are easier to place on your own. To place the cups, follow these steps.

1. It may be easiest to place the first cup on the back of the shoulder joint. To do this comfortably, take the cup in the opposite hand.
2. Reach across the chest and over the top of your shoulder joint so you don't have to torque your body too much. Place the cup on the back of the shoulder joint where you can reach the furthest without strain, optimally just above the crease where the backside of the armpit begins.

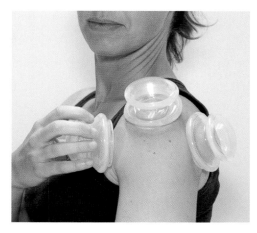

3. Place the next cup directly at the top of the joint, then work down the frontside of the joint, toward the armpit (see Steps 2 and 3 of "Stationary Cups, Supine Position" to find the exact location).
4. Place the last cup directly below the second cup, just ending where the armpit begins. This is where you will find the top of the humerus bone and the outermost point of the chest.
5. Allow cups to remain in place for a maximum of 3 minutes.
6. Remove cups one at a time. While it is recommended to remove cups in the order in which they were placed, this may be difficult to do to yourself, so remove cups from front to back.
7. Once cups have been removed, gently massage your shoulder joint for a few minutes for additional relief and recirculation.

Additional Application Option

See applications for stress relief and overall back tension and neck and shoulder tension on pages 135 to 143 for additional options for relief. The placement of cups around the entire joint will provide some relief, but when muscles that support the shoulder joint are holding additional tension to compensate for a compromised joint, more work may be required. When muscles compensate for a frozen shoulder joint, for example, you might see an imbalance of posture when someone is lifting something, using their whole torso instead of just their arms. In this case, the muscles of the neck, shoulders and back can be irritated from the frozen shoulder condition, too.

Elbow Problems

Elbow problems typically stem from inflammation that involves the tendons and associated muscles of the elbow joint. The most common among these is damage to or inflammation of the tendons in the elbow area, also known as tendinosis or tendonitis.

Most of the muscles in the upper extremity intersect with the elbow and can be affected. Lateral epicondylitis (tennis elbow) or medial epicondylitis (golfer's elbow) are terms often used to describe the pain in the elbow.

Causes

This type of pain is generally caused by repetitive motion injuries. Whether from work environments (computer work) or sports and exercise (golfer's or tennis elbow), elbow pain can vary from person to person. Inflammation usually starts in the muscle due to overuse and can lead to pain in the tendons or bones involved in the elbow joint.

Symptoms

Elbow pain can be sharp, dull, throbbing or aching. The elbow may feel stiff or "crunchy" as it moves through a range of motion, and the hand and wrist may feel weak.

Cups and Elbow Problems

The elbow joint is fairly awkward to apply cups to, but do not be discouraged. The negative pressure of cups is extremely effective to help relieve inflammation and tension in this small, tightly sensitive region. It is also recommended to treat the muscles that act on the joint, too, as they are involved in this condition.

Techniques

LIFT-AND-RELEASE APPLICATIONS can be applied all over the arm to help soften the tissue. This technique is especially helpful for initial applications directly at the elbow, where the tendons may be too sensitive for stationary cups.

MOVING CUPS along the entire arm may be soothing and offer much relief. Remember to use lighter suction pressure on the inside of the arm and to address the upper arm before working the lower arm to acknowledge the lymphatic system accordingly.

STATIONARY CUPS around the elbow can allow for an effective release of inflammation from the joint and involved tendons. Avoid strong suction on the inside of the forearm.

Conditions that may also benefit from these applications:

- Lateral epicondylitis (tennis elbow)
- Medial epicondylitis (golfer's elbow)
- Carpal tunnel syndrome

Primary Application

GENERAL ELBOW JOINT (STATIONARY CUPS, PRONE POSITION)

The prone position allows the best access to both sides of the elbow joint, with a relaxed arm extended over the side of table, as shown. Smaller cups work best, as the treatment area is small.

TARGET AREA INCLUDES: The elbow joint and attachment sites of flexor and extensor muscles of the wrist.

1
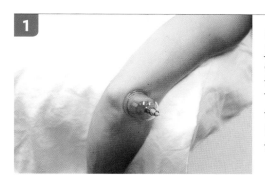

Place the first cup on the outside and on top of the elbow joint. To locate the starting point, place fingertips on the elbow bone (the olecranon process of the ulna bone in the forearm) and the thumb at the crease of the elbow joint. The cup should be placed in the space located between the fingers and thumb, directly over the top of the elbow joint. Be sure the cup is not over the soft space on the inside of the elbow; this is the antecubital endangerment site.

2
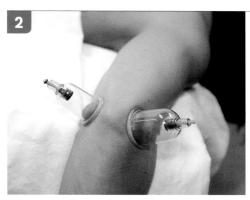

Place the second cup directly opposite the first cup on the inside of the elbow joint. To locate the starting point, use the same location instructions as described in Step 1, placing the cup in between the elbow and inner crease. There will be a small bone about 2 fingers' width away (diagonally) from the elbow bone; this is the medial epicondyle of the humerus. Be sure the cup is just below this second bone to the best of your ability.

Note

It is best to use lighter suction here. Be mindful of any "nervy" or tingly sensations, as this may indicate that you are irritating various nerves (radial, median, ulnar) that pass through the area. Remove and reapply if this happens, making sure this sensation is not felt when the cup is attached.

EXAMPLE
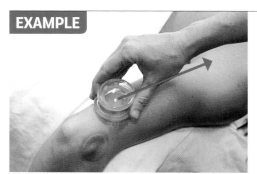

In this case, the person suffers from tendonitis, carpal tunnel syndrome and general elbow pain. Notice the red cup mark? The person immediately said her elbow felt "softer and less tight."

RECOMMENDED AFTER STATIONARY CUPS HAVE BEEN REMOVED: Use either your hand or a cup to lightly encourage recirculation.

Optional Applications

TRICEPS BRACHII MUSCLE (STATIONARY CUPS, PRONE POSITION)

The triceps brachii muscle attaches to the elbow bone (the olecranon process of the ulna bone) and its tightness can often contribute to a lot of pain on the elbow. Be sure the arm is relaxed, extended off the side of table, as shown. This application requires 3 or 4 cups, depending on the length of the upper arm.

TARGET AREA INCLUDES: The triceps brachii and posterior deltoid muscles.

1. Apply the first cup directly above the elbow bone in the center of the triceps muscle. The edge of the cup should be just above the bone.
2. Place the second cup directly above the first cup, progressing along the center line of the upper arm, toward the shoulder.
3. Place the third cup directly above the second cup, continuing toward the shoulder.
4. Place the last cup directly above the third cup, secured at the top of the arm, just above the armpit.
5. Allow cups to remain in place for a maximum of 3 minutes but no less than 30 seconds.
6. Remove the cups one at a time, in the order they were applied for the best relief.

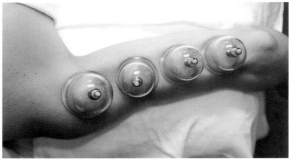
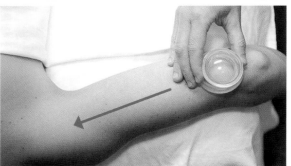

> Conditions that may also benefit from this application:
>
> - Triceps tendonitis
> - General tightness in triceps area

RECOMMENDED AFTER STATIONARY CUPS HAVE BEEN REMOVED: Use either your hand or a cup to lightly encourage recirculation. Use either the moving or lift-and-release technique, depending on sensitivity.

The direction of movement is up the arm, toward the armpit. This line of movement may be repeated a few times.

LATERAL ELBOW PAIN (STATIONARY CUPS, SUPINE POSITION)

▸ Depending on the pain areas and symptoms, apply 2 smaller cups above and below the elbow joint and address it indirectly (below, left).
▸ Touch with the fingers to see where more tightness is felt and place cups there.
▸ Allow to remain in place for a maximum of 3 minutes but no less than 30 seconds.
▸ Remove cups one at a time, in the order they were applied for the best relief.

Conditions that may also benefit from this application:

• Lateral epicondylitis (tennis elbow)
• Carpal tunnel syndrome
• General elbow stiffness

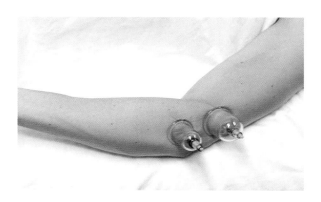
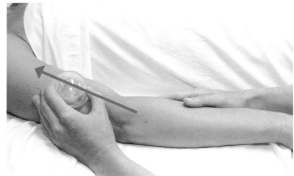

RECOMMENDED AFTER STATIONARY CUPS HAVE BEEN REMOVED: Use either your hand or a cup to lightly encourage recirculation (above, right). Use either the moving or lift-and-release technique, depending on sensitivity. The direction of movement is up the arm, toward the armpit. This line of movement may be repeated a few times.

SELF-CARE APPLICATION

Any of the applications noted in the optional applications may be chosen for self-care. The seated position is best, with the arm resting comfortably on a table or pillow. Smaller silicone cups seem to work best for applying them on your own in this area. Using the free hand, the silicone cups are easy to apply and remove while the treated arm is resting.

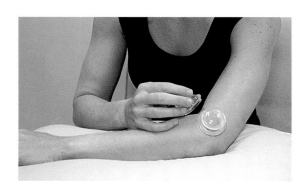

Carpal Tunnel Syndrome

The carpal tunnel is a narrow passageway of bones and ligaments where the median nerve and tendons run through the wrist. Any compression or entrapment of the median nerve as it passes through the retinaculum (a thick band of connective tissue that helps to keep tendons and muscles in place) of the wrist will result in carpal tunnel syndrome, a condition that causes pain, numbness and tingling in the wrist, hand and fingers.

Causes

Carpal tunnel syndrome can be caused by a wide variety of contributing factors: congenital predisposition (a naturally smaller carpal tunnel space); injury to the wrist that leaves scar tissue; repetitive motion, such as computer work or hairstyling; or other underlying health conditions, such as diabetes or rheumatoid arthritis.

Symptoms

Symptoms may include numbness, tingling or itching of the hand, thumb and most fingers. It can cause the hand to feel weak or swollen, even if there is no swelling present. This sensation can sometimes worsen while sleeping, when wrists are in a flexed, curled position.

Carpal tunnel-like symptoms can often be confused with carpal tunnel syndrome. A number of contributing factors could create similar pain sensations; for example, if there is compression, impingements or kinks in other nerves, such as the radial and ulnar nerve, that branch off the brachial plexus in the upper extremity (see Anatomy FYI, opposite page).

A person with carpal tunnel syndrome can often have multiple surgeries, but the pain still persists.

Cupping and Carpal Tunnel Syndrome

Cups can be applied in many ways to help relieve carpal tunnel syndrome or similar symptoms. Because of their decompressive nature, cups are very effective in lifting and separating the soft tissues that may be compressed and thus add to the nerve's irritation. Cups can also bring fluid into the more delicate, avascular tendons (less blood supply than muscles) in the carpal tunnel region.

Face cups, in particular, work well in the carpal tunnel area because of their small sizes and better control of lighter suction.

Conditions that may also benefit from these applications:

- Thoracic outlet syndrome
- Bursitis
- Tendonitis
- Elbow problems
- General arm tightness

Note

Working directly in the carpal tunnel can be dangerous because of the many arteries and veins that pass through near the surface of the skin. Any cups applied here should be controlled with lighter suction. Also, any stationary cups on the anterior (inside) of the forearm should be applied comfortably and for short periods. Lift-and-release cups or moving cups with lighter suction are preferred for the inside of the forearm, from wrist to elbow. Be especially cautious if there is a clotting potential or if person is taking blood thinners.

Techniques

LIFT-AND-RELEASE APPLICATIONS on the entire upper extremity can be very effective and quite comfortable if the arm is especially sensitive to initial applications. This can be especially helpful on the anterior upper arm and forearm, where vascular bodies are more superficial.

MOVING CUPS can be sensitive, so start light and work into stronger pressure if desired and tolerated.

STATIONARY CUPS can be placed along the entire arm. Because of the vascular considerations on the inside of the arm, work stationary cups along the outside of the arm to be safe.

BEFORE YOU BEGIN: Carpal tunnel syndrome is predominantly a one-sided ailment, and these applications should therefore be used to treat the affected side. If symptoms are bilateral (in both arms), however, then you may choose to treat both arms. Address one entire arm first, then the other arm.

Note

There are no primary applications for carpal tunnel syndrome since each person displays different symptoms. Assess individual discomforts and apply cups accordingly. If a person feels pain along the outside of the upper arm and chest region, for example, choose the appropriate option below.

Anatomy FYI

The Brachial Plexus is a bundle of nerves that innervates the upper extremity. It begins in the neck, passes through the Thoracic Outlet in the upper chest and shoulder, and then divides into the radial, median, and ulnar nerves before continuing down the length of the arm.)

Optional Applications

ENTIRE ARM (LIFT-AND-RELEASE OR MOVING CUPS, SUPINE OR PRONE POSITION)

- If treating the inside of the arm, prone is the best position.
- If treating the outside of the arm, supine is the best position.

This application of cups is used to encourage lymphatic drainage and overall circulation of the entire upper extremity, which can help alleviate carpal tunnel discomfort. Such an application is also an effective way to treat the entire upper arm when stationary cups are uncomfortable. See Chapter 9, page 214, for detailed, step-by-step instructions on how to address the entire arm in this manner.

UPPER ARM (STATIONARY CUPS, SUPINE POSITION)

TARGET AREA INCLUDES: Portions of the biceps brachii, triceps brachii, coracobrachialis, middle and anterior deltoid, pectoralis major muscles and into the bicipital groove.

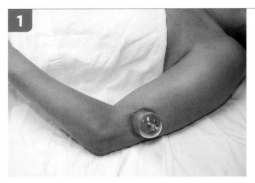

1 Place the first cup just above the elbow joint. To locate the starting point, place the fingertips in the crease of the elbow, arm slightly bent to relax tendons around elbow. Slide the fingers straight out to the outside of the arm, approximately 4 fingers' width, and make contact with the elbow bone (the olecranon process of the ulna). Place the cup just above this line marked by your fingers, in the center of the arm's soft tissue space. In this example, the first cup is placed approximately 2 fingers' width above this marked line, due to the size of the arm.

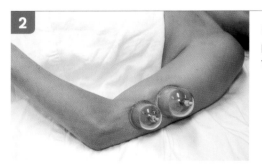

2 Place the second cup directly above the first cup, progressing up the center line of the outer arm toward the shoulder.

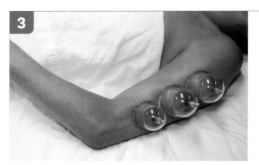

3 Place the third cup directly above the second cup, continuing up the center line of the outer arm.

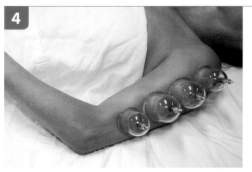

4 Place the fourth cup directly above the third cup; this should be positioned in the deltoid muscles, about one hand's width below the actual shoulder joint in the centerline of the outer arm.

The cup will be placed just below the shoulder joint when in the correct location; it should not be covering the shoulder joint directly.

5

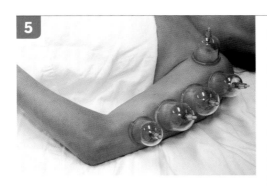

Note

Remember this is a sensitive area for blood vessels and nerves, so strong suction should not be used here. Be mindful of any "nervy" or tingly sensations, as this may indicate an irritation of various nerves that pass through the area. Remove and reapply cups if this happens, making sure this sensation is not felt when the cup is reattached.

Place the last cup just next to the fourth cup, approximately 1 to 2 fingers' width apart, depending on the size of the person's shoulder, going in toward the chest. This placement will cover the bicipital groove, which will feel like a tight muscle band in the front of the shoulder joint.

To locate it, place the fingertips at the top crease of the armpit. Lightly slide the fingers straight up toward the top of the shoulder joint. A short distance up, approximately 3 fingers' width, begin to lightly rub up and down with the fingertips to feel for a tight band of muscle that travels across the front of the shoulder. This band, which will include the bicipital tendon, is the location to place the last cup, directly over the front of the shoulder joint. The cup will be equidistant between the crease of the armpit and the very top of the shoulder when in the correct location.

Allow cups to remain in place for a maximum of 3 minutes but no less than 30 seconds. Remove cups one at a time, in the order they were applied for the best relief.

RECOMMENDED AFTER STATIONARY CUPS HAVE BEEN REMOVED: Use either your hand or a cup to lightly encourage recirculation.

Anatomy FYI

The bicipital groove is a bony landmark on the humerus (on the upper arm) where the pectoralis major, teres major and latissimus dorsi muscles attach. The biceps brachii, coracobrachialis and anterior deltoid muscles, as well as the brachial plexus and major arteries and veins of the upper extremities, pass through this region.

LOWER ARM (STATIONARY CUPS, SUPINE POSITION)

This application should be applied only after working the upper arm, working the proximal part of the arm before the distal to encourage lymphatic drainage.

TARGET AREA INCLUDES: The extensor muscles of the forearm.

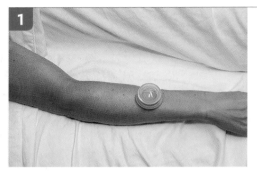

Place the first cup slightly above the wrist joint. To locate the starting point, place the fingers on the back of the wrist. The cup should be placed about one hand's width above the fold of the wrist, in the center line of the arm, for the most comfortable location. Trying to place a cup directly on the back of the wrist may be challenging due to the bony structures and superficial blood vessels.

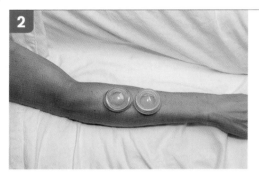

Place the second cup directly above the first cup, progressing up the forearm toward the elbow.

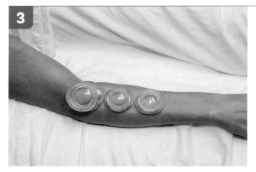

Place the last cup directly above the second cup, ending at the elbow joint. While exact locations may vary, the last cup should end at the elbow joint. Allow cups to remain in place for a maximum of 3 minutes but no less than a minimum of 30 seconds. Remove cups one at a time, in the order they were applied for the best relief.

RECOMMENDED AFTER STATIONARY CUPS HAVE BEEN REMOVED: Use either your hand or a cup to lightly encourage recirculation.

ANTERIOR (INSIDE) FOREARM (STATIONARY CUPS, PRONE POSITION)

When trying to apply stationary cups to the inside of the arm, it is important that the arm is fully relaxed. When applying cups, instruct the person to assume the prone position with their arm along the side of the body.

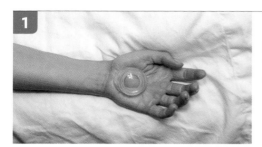

1 Place the first cup in the center of the palm of the hand, between the wrist and the fingertips. Be sure not to place the cup directly in the crease of the wrist, where there are exposed blood vessels and nerves.

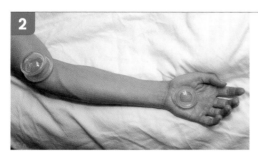

2 Place the second cup over the elbow joint. To locate it, place the fingertips on the two pointed bones located at the elbow joint. Place the cup gently over or in between these bones, depending on the size of the joint (see Safety Point, below).

In this example, notice how the cup is placed above the superficial blood vessel, not on top of it.

Allow cups to remain in place for a maximum of 3 minutes but no less than 30 seconds.

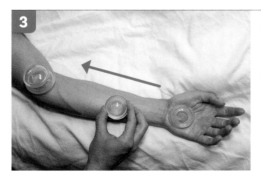

3 While the two cups remain in place, you may use 1 additional cup to treat the inside of the forearm. Rather than place stationary cups over this delicate vascular region, use the lift-and-release technique or a gentle moving cup in this area. The area to treat begins just above the wrist crease and works up toward the second cup, which remains at the elbow joint.

To measure a safe place to begin, place 3 middle fingers (not the pinky or thumb) just below where the wrist folds. Just above where the third finger rests is where the cup should start to be used. This line of movement may be repeated a few times while the other two cups are attached. Remove cups one at a time, in the order they were applied for the best relief.

Safety Point
....

This location has superficially exposed blood vessels and nerves, so strong suction pressure should not be used here. Also, no stationary cups should be placed directly on the forearm between the elbow and wrist — such an application could potentially cause harm to the vessels in close proximity. Rather, a moving cup or lift-and-release application from the wrist to the elbow will work best to address this area. (See Chapter 5: "Safe Cupping" for more information about such vascular considerations.)

SELF-CARE APPLICATION

Silicone cups are better than the manual pump gun here, since you would need both hands to work the pump gun and maneuver cups, while silicone cups are easy to squeeze and apply with one hand. The arm you are working on should be relaxed and supported.

1. Best applied in a seated position, with arm resting comfortably on a table or pillow.
2. Follow stationary cup placement in Steps 1 and 2 (supine position). If applying stationary cups, place the cups along the back of your arm, progressing along the center line of the arm as detailed in previous optional applications, page 160.
3. If applying cups on the inside of your forearm, work up the length of the arm from the wrist toward the elbow, using lighter suction with an optional stationary cup to your palm, page 161.

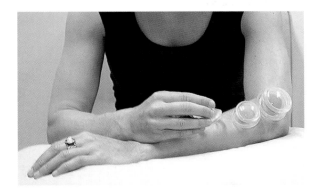

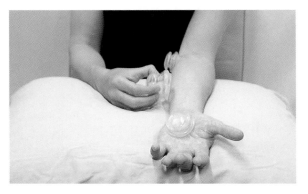

Additional Application Options

Consider the applications mentioned in the sections on elbow problems, starting on page 152, and neck and shoulder tension, starting on page 138, for additional applications that address carpal tunnel syndrome symptoms.

Sciatica

The sciatic nerve is the largest and longest nerve in the body. It begins in the lower spine, then travels through the pelvis, continues under the piriformis muscle in the buttock/gluteal region and down into the thigh, where it splits into two nerve branches (the tibial and peroneal nerves) behind the knee to innervate muscles of the lower leg and foot.

Causes

Sciatica (lumbar radiculopathy) is not a condition but rather a descriptive symptom of more significant underlying conditions. Causes may include vertebral disc compression, a herniated lumbar disc, pregnancy or spinal injury. Piriformis syndrome can have symptoms similar to sciatica but is more a condition of spasm and muscular compression of the piriformis muscle, which can irritate the sciatic nerve and have pain patterns similar to true sciatica.

Symptoms

Symptoms may be infrequent or constant, and symptoms can vary based on the location of nerve impingement. Examples of symptoms include constant pain in one buttock or leg (rarely both sides), pain that worsens when sitting, leg pain described as burning or tingling (instead of a dull ache), weakness, or numbness.

Cupping and Sciatica

Because of the decompressive nature of cupping, this is a beneficial therapy to relieve pressure and pain associated with sciatica. Light, dispersing cupping can soothe any superficial irritation, especially when sitting adds pressure to an already compressed region. Working deeper into the musculature, stationary cups can allow for the slow softening of the tight tissue and encourage the involved areas to release their tension as the cups sit in place for a few minutes at relevant locations. Be sure to palpate and assess for areas that feel tighter than others — that's where you'll want to place the cups.

Techniques

THE LIFT-AND-RELEASE TECHNIQUE is a great introductory application, especially if stationary cups are too intense at first.

MOVING CUPS with lighter pressure can prove very beneficial in both the gluteal and hip region. Be mindfully of any referral pains and always work within one's comfort.

STATIONARY CUPS can be placed strategically wherever pain may be concentrated or tighter tissue is palpated.

Conditions that may also benefit from these applications:

- Bursitis
- Arthritis
- Restless leg syndrome
- General hip tension
- Fibromyalgia (symptomatic in the hip and gluteal region)

DID YOU KNOW?

The sciatic nerve is actually made up of five different nerves, which originate from the lumbar spine (L4 and L5) and the first three segments of the sacral spine (S1, S2 and S3) before joining together to continue down into the leg. It can be about the thickness of a human thumb at its largest point, located in the gluteal region.

Primary Application

SCIATICA (STATIONARY CUPS, PRONE POSITION)

POSITION OPTION: Lying on one side allows easy access to this area, whether for applying cups to another person (if lying on their stomach is uncomfortable) or for self-care. See the self-care application, opposite page.

TARGET AREA INCLUDES: The SI joint, portions of the gluteal muscles and the piriformis muscle.

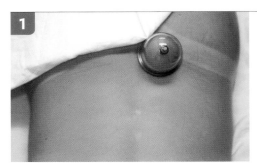

1

In this example, the left hip is being treated.

Place the first cup over the SI joint. To locate it, place the fingertips at the base of spine where it meets the tailbone (sacrum). Slowly move the fingers a very short distance out — in this case to the left — approximately 2 fingers' width, toward the side of the body. There will be a small divot; this is the SI joint. Apply the first cup here. The cup should not be directly over the spine when attached.

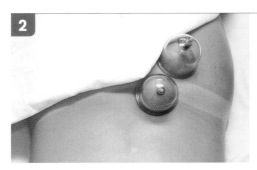

2

Place the second cup just below and to the side, about 1 finger's width down and the same amount diagonally between the first cup and the hip joint. Apply the cup directly over the attachment of the piriformis muscle, to the side of the sacrum.

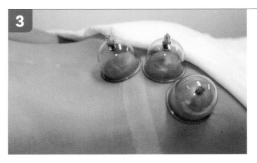

3

Place the third cup directly below the second cup, following a diagonal line from the second cup toward the hip joint.

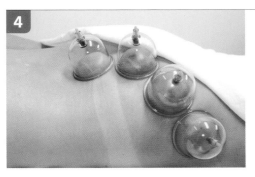

4

Place the last cup below the third cup, continuing in a diagonal line toward the hip joint. Apply it directly over the hip joint.

Use your fingers to lightly feel for the joint. If you are having difficulty finding the spot, slowly twist the leg in and out a little — you will feel the femur bone in the joint rub under your fingers as the leg moves.

Allow cups to remain in place for a maximum of 3 minutes but no less than a minimum of 30 seconds. Remove cups one at a time, in the order they were applied for the best relief.

Optional Applications

GLUTEAL REGION (MOVING CUP, PRONE POSITION)

Applying a moving cup following stationary cups can be very effective. (Moving cups can also work well as a stand-alone application.) After placing and removing stationary cups, this not only encourages the movement of blood and lymph through the hip, but it also allows the person to feel for any tight areas that may still persist in the hip. Moving cups also help loosen the overall gluteal region, especially if stationary cups are uncomfortable.

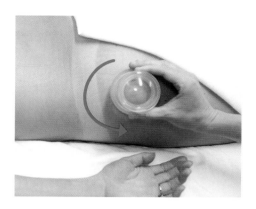

TARGET AREA INCLUDES: The entire gluteal hip region — all gluteus and deep lateral rotator muscles.

▸ Begin with a lighter suction; as the tissue softens, you may increase pressure if desired.

▸ Attach the cup lightly in the center of the gluteal region, then gently lift it away from the hip until you feel a slight tension engage.

▸ Next, slide the cup around the entire hip region in a circular motion (clockwise or counterclockwise). You may choose to do larger or smaller circles, depending on the contours of the body and the comfort of the recipient.

▸ These circular movements may be repeated a few times. If it feels good, you may work this area for a few minutes (recommended to a maximum of 3 minutes, just as with the stationary cups). Do not overwork the area.

SCIATICA COMPENSATION, OPPOSITE HIP

While sciatica may be symptomatic in one hip, the other hip should also be addressed with some bodywork, whether repeating the Primary Application (optional moving cups), or even without cups (hands-on manual therapy). This is not only because the other hip may overcompensate for the affected hip, but also to help maintain balance in the sacrum and pelvis. Given the musculature in the pelvis, working only half of the area could leave the other hip feeling tighter.

SELF-CARE APPLICATION

Lying down on your side works best here, as long as there are no discomforts or symptoms. Place a pillow under the head for support, knees bent slightly toward the torso (as shown). You should also work both sides on yourself.

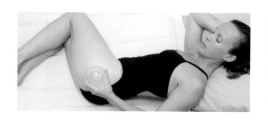

IT Band Restrictions

The iliotibial (IT) band is a long band of connective tissue that runs along the outside of the thigh. It is a common attachment site for many muscles in the gluteal, hip and thigh region, and connects to the lower leg just below the knee joint. The IT band both stabilizes and supports the various movements of the hip and knee joints.

Causes

This area can be easily irritated from excess use and tension and create a great deal of discomfort. Sports or exercise (for example, running and cycling), in particular, cause tension in the IT band because so many leg muscles are connected to it. Postural imbalances (pelvic distortions, scoliosis) can also cause the IT band to become more restricted. Stretching the muscles in the lower extremities is good practice — even a necessity — to keep the IT band from becoming too tight.

Symptoms

Considering the role and articulations of the IT band, pain may be felt in the knee, hip or side of the leg. There may be localized inflammation in the lateral knee, a stinging or tingling pain along the outside of the leg, or difficulty walking or performing other movements if left untreated. Such symptoms can also be related to sciatica.

Cupping and IT Band Restrictions

Cupping draws fluid into this region with relatively minimal blood supply, making the IT band softer and more flexible to encourage ease of movement. Cupping here can be compared to the effects of foam-rolling the leg out; however, the negative pressure of cupping "rolls" it out with the greater benefit of lifting and stretching without pressing on an already tight area.

Techniques

LIFT-AND-RELEASE APPLICATIONS can be used as initial applications to help loosen this tight area. Work up the leg from the outside of the knee toward the hip joint.

MOVING CUPS can be used to soften the IT band, working from the knee to the hip if the area is too sensitive for stationary cups.

STATIONARY CUPS can be applied to the IT band. The tighter the IT band, however, the more challenging this application may be. Cups may pop off or not take hold if the band is too tight.

Conditions and areas that may also benefit from these applications:

- Bursitis
- General hip discomforts
- Knee problems

Primary Application

IT BAND (STATIONARY CUPS, SUPINE POSITION)

TARGET AREA INCLUDES: The majority of the IT band and portions of the tensor fasciae latae muscle and attachments of hip muscles at the hip joint.

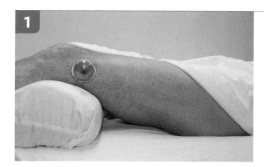

1 Place the first cup above the knee joint, in the center of the outer thigh. To locate the starting point, find the kneecap (patella). The location varies from person to person (for example, with a thicker thigh), but the average spacing is approximately 2 fingers' width away from the side of the top of the kneecap. This is the spot where the first cup should be placed.

The exact insertion of the IT band is just below the knee on the tibia. Cups can be placed there, too, but the bony location may make this challenging.

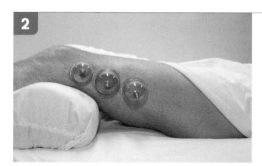

2 Place the second cup directly above the first one, progressing up the center of the outer thigh. Continue placing cups up the entire length of the outer thigh, with the third cup directly following the second cup, edge to edge.

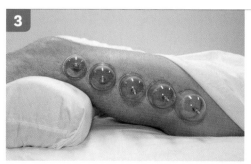

3 Continue the application process — placing the fourth cup next to the third one, then the fifth and sixth cup, etc., until you reach the hip joint (where the femur inserts into the hip).

To locate the hip joint, locate the crease at the front of the hip with your fingertips, then slide the fingers out and around to the side of the hip where the joint is.

If you are having difficulty finding the spot, slowly twist the leg in and out a little. You will feel the femur bone in the joint rub under your fingers as the leg moves. This is the hip joint.

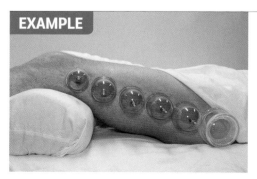

EXAMPLE In this case, the person has a very long thigh, so 6 cups were required. Notice the large silicone cup at the top, which can be used in place of plastic cups if you require more cups to cover a large area.

Allow cups to remain in place for a maximum of 3 minutes but no less than a minimum of 30 seconds. Remove cups one at a time, in the order in which they were applied for the best relief.

RECOMMENDED AFTER STATIONARY CUPS HAVE BEEN REMOVED: Use either your hand or a cup to lightly encourage recirculation.

Optional Applications

IT BAND (MOVING CUPS)

Applying a moving cup following stationary cups can be very effective. (Moving cups can also work well as a stand-alone application.) After placing and removing stationary cups, applying a moving cup not only encourages the movement of blood and lymph through the leg, but also allows the person applying the cups to feel for any restrictions. As the cup slides along the IT band, working from the knee to the hip, you will be able to feel the tissue "crackle" or

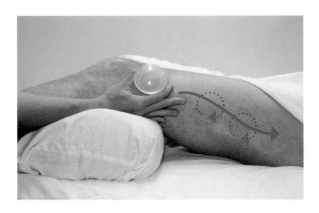

"crunch" through the cup, highlighting the restrictions in the IT band. Tissue will slowly soften with each pass, bringing immediate relief and change. Be sure to lift the cup as you slide it along. Follow these steps:

- ▸ Begin with a lighter suction; as the tissue softens, you may increase pressure if desired.
- ▸ Attach the cup lightly, then gently lift it away from the thigh until you feel a slight tension engage.
- ▸ Then slide the cup up the outside of the thigh toward the hip joint.
- ▸ This line of movement (from the side of knee, up the outside of the thigh, ending at the hip joint) may be repeated a few times. If it feels good, you may work this area for a few minutes (recommended to a maximum of 3 minutes, just as with stationary cups). Do not overwork the area.

You can twist the cup in your hand as you move it up the leg, which can feel very soothing, similar to the kneading sensation you feel when a therapist manipulates the IT band with the hands. Attach the cup to the skin, lift it gently away from the thigh until you feel tension engage, then twist your hand back and forth as you go or use full rotations of the cup (like turning on a faucet), whichever you prefer.

ALTERNATIVE: LIFT-AND-RELEASE TECHNIQUE

If sliding in this area is uncomfortable, use the lift-and-release technique until the tissue is softer and more responsive to moving cups.

Safety Point

While cupping is effective on the legs, remember not to use cups directly over any varicose veins, to avoid further damage. (See Chapter 5: "Safe Cupping" for more information.)

MUSCLES OF THE THIGH

The same methods of application that are used for the IT band can also be used for all muscles of the thigh.

- Quadriceps (front of thigh)
- Hamstrings (back of thigh)
- Adductors (inside of thigh)

SELF-CARE APPLICATION

Lying down (preferably on one side, legs slightly bent, as shown), start by placing cups at your hip joint. I find it easier to begin placing stationary cups at my hip joint, then work down to the knee are far as I can comfortably go. If using moving cups, I can easily reach down toward the outside of the knee and slide the cup up toward my hip in this position, bending knees up closer if needed to reach comfortably. You

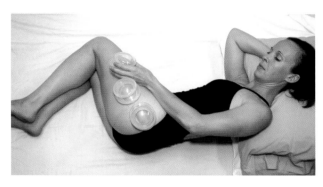

may choose any previously mentioned applications (stationary cups are shown here). To place the stationary cups on your own, follow these steps:

1. To locate the hip joint, use your fingertips to find the outermost part of your hip bones (where you typically place your hands on your hip when standing), then walk your fingers straight down the body toward the leg until you feel your femur bone in the middle of the hip. To be sure of the proper location, twist your leg a little inward and then outward — the femur bone will move in the joint under your fingers. The hip joint will be about one hand's width below your side hip bone (where you may rest your hand's when standing), and this is the location of your first cup.
2. Place the first cup directly over the hip joint and then place the cups edge to edge along your IT band, working your way down the center line of your outer thigh, toward the knee. Keep your legs in a bent position to make it easier to reach and position cups closer to your knee without too much adjustment.
3. Allow cups to remain on for a maximum of 3 minutes, but no less than 30 seconds.
4. Remove cups one at a time, in the order they were placed for the best relief.
5. Once cups have been removed, it is highly recommended to use a moving cup along the IT band (working up the leg, from the knee toward the hip) to encourage recirculation. This moving cup may also allow you to feel for any restrictions or to encourage more softening of the IT band. Twist the cup as you slide it along for an added sensation of loosening.

Knee Problems

The knee is a very complex yet vulnerable joint. There are technically two joints here: the gliding joint of the patella and femur (the patellofemoral joint) and the hinge joint of the femur and the tibia (the tibiofemoral joint). The kneecap, or patella bone, protects the knee joint. The quadriceps tendon envelops the patella as it connects the thigh to the tibia. Within the knee joint are many tendons and ligaments that keep the whole structure together.

Causes

Knee pain can be caused by a multitude of contributing factors, such as sprains, strains, overuse or dislocation. Conditions such as tendonitis, bursitis, osteoarthritis, a torn meniscus or ligament damage can contribute to short- or long-term knee problems.

Other factors include injury (even worse if not treated), improper body mechanics, poor posture, not stretching leg muscles before or after physical exertion or being overweight. Torn or damaged tissue is common in the knee joint.

Symptoms

Pain can be long-lasting or acute (temporary), dull and aching or sharp and shooting; swelling may exist; there may be a limited function or range of motion (the knee could "lock" straight or, if bent, it may be difficult to straighten completely). More intense knee pain should be diagnosed medically as soon as possible.

Cupping and the Knee

Cups can help draw out chronic inflammation from the knee joint, as well as help soften and loosen the region, especially when the knee feels tight. Be sure to **never** place a cup directly over a swollen knee, as this would cause further harm. (See "Working with Inflammation" in Chapter 10 for more information.)

Techniques

THE LIFT-AND-RELEASE TECHNIQUE is effective for initial applications here or when the area is too sensitive to use stationary cups.

MOVING CUPS do not work well for direct knee pain because of the bony structures. Instead, consider using moving cups above the knee in the quadriceps muscles or along the IT band to loosen them.

STATIONARY CUPS applied directly on either side of the knee joint are effective for drawing out chronic inflammation. Be sure that the suction is not too strong here. The more painful the knee, the weaker the suction should be.

> ### DID YOU KNOW?
>
> For every pound (0.5 kg) a person is overweight, the knee must absorb an additional 4 pounds (2 kg) of pressure.

Primary Applications

KNEE JOINT DIRECTLY (STATIONARY CUPS, SUPINE POSITION)

This application is good for knee joints that are not compromised or damaged (for example, a torn meniscus). Silicone cups are used for this demonstration. They are typically more comfortable when applied directly on bony landmarks and make it easier to produce successful suction connections when bony landmarks don't offer a flat surface for manual plastic (or glass) cups.

TARGET AREA INCLUDES: The knee joint, ligaments (LCL, or lateral collateral ligament, and MCL, or medial collateral ligament) and lowest portion of the IT band.

BEFORE YOU BEGIN: Be sure that the knee is fully supported and relaxed; place a pillow or cushion behind the knee joint for the best support.

Safety Point

Make sure there are no torn or damaged ligaments or tendons in the knee joint before attempting this application.

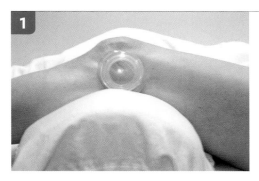

1 Place the first cup directly on the outside of the knee joint next to the patella (kneecap). To locate the starting point, place the fingers on top of the kneecap. Slowly move the fingers in a straight line down the side of the knee to the back of the knee, where the crease begins. The cup should be placed in the space between those two spots. If you are having difficulty finding this spot, slightly bend the knee and straighten it to find that middle "hinge" point between the kneecap and the back of the knee.

Do not press the cup into the skin while trying to attach it, or it could be painful.

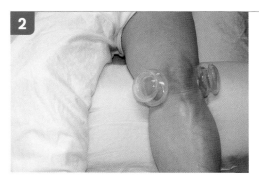

2 Place the second cup on the inside of the knee, directly opposite where the first cup was placed. If this spot is difficult to locate, draw the same line from the top of kneecap straight down to the inside crease of the knee. Place the cup in the space between those two points.

Allow cups to remain in place for a maximum of 3 minutes but no less than a minimum of 30 seconds. Remove cups one at a time, in the order they were applied for the best relief.

RECOMMENDED AFTER STATIONARY CUPS HAVE BEEN REMOVED: Use either your hand or a cup to lightly encourage recirculation.

Optional Application

DIRECTLY ABOVE THE KNEE (STATIONARY OR MOVING CUP, SUPINE POSITION)

This application is a good option for indirectly addressing the knee joint if any potentially damaged structures exist (such as a torn meniscus) or if direct application to knee joint is uncomfortable.

TARGET AREA INCLUDES: The quadriceps tendon and patellar (kneecap) tendon.

BEFORE YOU BEGIN: Be sure that the knee is fully supported and relaxed; place a pillow or cushion behind the knee joint for best support.

STATIONARY CUP OPTION: Apply 1 stationary cup directly above the knee joint to address the quadriceps tendon that encases the patella (kneecap) bone.

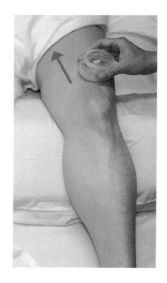

▸ Allow this single cup to remain in place for a maximum of 3 minutes but no less than a minimum of 30 seconds.
▸ Remove this cup, then follow with a few strokes of a moving cup up the thigh, toward the groin, to lightly encourage recirculation.

MOVING CUP OPTION: Using a moving cup along the length of the quadriceps (also contributes to softening of the quadriceps tendon/patellar ligament and easing tension on the knee joint).

The starting point is just above the kneecap, and the line of movement travels along the length of the thigh, ending below the front hip crease region.

SELF-CARE APPLICATION

Applying cups to your own knee is very easy. Whichever application you choose, be sure that you are seated and fully resting your knee, preferably with your leg extended in front of you and a pillow behind the knee for support. You may use silicone cups (demonstrated here) or manual cups for either of the suggested applications for knee problems.

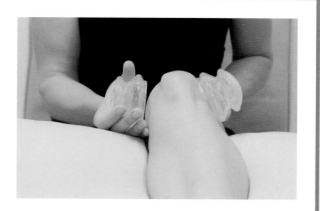

Plantar Fasciitis

Plantar fasciitis, literally meaning inflammation of the plantar fascia, is a condition with pain at the bottom of your foot, often more near the heel. The plantar fascia is a band of connective tissue that runs along the bottom of the foot from your heel bone to the ball of your foot, and it provides shock absorption as well as support for the arch. Repetitive micro-tearing of the plantar fascia can cause inflammation, which may remain in the tissue and prolong the discomfort of the already tight and painful plantar fascia and lead to further pain associated with this condition.

Causes

Plantar fasciitis can be caused by a number of factors, including the start or sudden change of an exercise program, wearing bad or non-supportive shoes, prolonged lack of use or inactivity, pregnancy and lack of flexibility in the lower leg, calf and foot muscles.

Symptoms

Plantar fasciitis symptoms predominantly involve pain anywhere along the bottom of the foot, especially around the heel, where the plantar fascia originates. The pain can be more intense during the first steps of the day or after long periods of walking, running or hiking. This pain can also be brought on by initial steps after lack of mobility for long periods (bedridden), being overweight or throughout pregnancy.

Cupping and Plantar Fasciitis

Cups are a welcome treatment because they can take effect with negative pressure rather than pressing on the already very tight and restricted tissue. The release of embedded inflammation is also a great benefit. Using moving cups along the lower leg toward the knee will encourage lymph drainage of any released inflammation but will also address potentially tight muscles.

Techniques

LIFT-AND-RELEASE APPLICATIONS are effective for initial applications in the entire region. You can even "pop" the cup off the bottom of the foot for an added stimulating sensation.

MOVING CUPS work well on the bottom of the foot; that is, if you can get a cup to slide and the foot is big enough. Moving cups also help to address the entire lower limb.

STATIONARY CUPS help slowly release tight tissue wherever they are placed. They also work well to draw fluids into these small, often dehydrated and tight areas.

Conditions that may also benefit from these applications:

- Neuropathy (monitor sensitivity to pressure)
- Achilles tendonitis
- Morton's neuroma (thickened nerve tissue, in between the 2nd and 3rd or 3rd and 4th metatarsal bones, just below the toes in the ball of the foot)
- Generally tight calf and foot muscles

Primary Application

BOTTOM OF THE FOOT (STATIONARY CUPS, PRONE POSITION)

Silicone cups are used in these applications as they tend to work best on the foot. You can even press *into* the cup while it is being held against the bottom of the foot to help it attach if you are having difficulty. Silicone cups generally mold to the curves of the foot better than the manual pump gun cups do, too.

TARGET AREA INCLUDES: The plantar fascia and flexor muscles of the foot.

BEFORE YOU BEGIN: Make sure that the foot is fully supported and relaxed; place a pillow or cushion under the front of the foot and ankle for best support. Apply oil or cream liberally — you may not be able to cup the foot tissues that are drier or more callused.

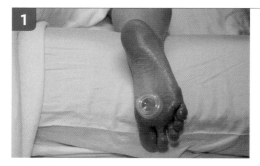

Place the first cup directly under the toes, on the ball of the foot just before it dips into the arch of the foot; this is where the distal end of the plantar fascia attaches.

Generally, the most common line of tension is just below the second and big toe (as shown). However, if the person feels more tension along another line on the bottom of the foot (for example, closer to the smallest toe), then follow these instructions beginning below the appropriate toe.

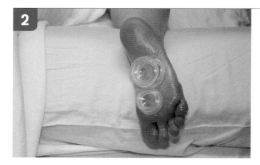

Place the second cup directly beside the first cup, in the arch of the foot, progressing toward the heel.

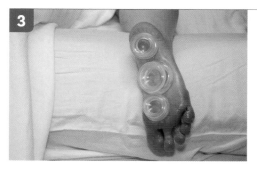

Place the last cup on the heel itself; this is where the plantar fascia begins and where pain is often more prominent.

If the foot is large, you may be able to attach 3 or 4 small to medium-sized cups (2 or 3 smaller-sized cups for smaller feet). Do the best you can to improvise according to the person's foot size.

Allow cups to remain for a maximum of 3 minutes but no less than a minimum of 30 seconds. Remove cups one at a time, in the order they were applied for the best relief.

Optional Application

ADDED STATIONARY CUPS TO CALF MUSCLES, PRONE POSITION

Any tight calf muscles can contribute to tightness in the foot, so it might be beneficial to add treatment with stationary cups to the lower limb.

TARGET AREA INCLUDES: Portions of the Achilles tendon and gastrocnemius, soleus (calf) and plantaris muscles.

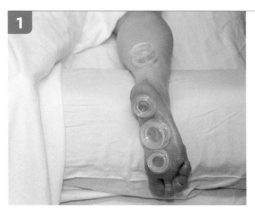

1 Place a pillow under the front of the foot for support. While stationary cups are still in place at the bottom of the foot (Primary Application), continue applying cups up the calf. Pay attention to the length of time it takes to continue applying these cups so you limit the time cups are placed on the foot.

Place a cup at the Achilles tendon, located just proximal to the heel bone at the lowest part of the calf muscle. It may be difficult to attach a cup here, so place a cup just above it, which will also be beneficial.

To locate this point, walk the fingertips from the heel straight up into the calf area. Place a cup on the first area you feel with soft tissue where a cup can be attached comfortably, about one hand's width above the heel; this will be at the top of the Achilles tendon. The calf area can be very sensitive, so be sure to begin with lighter suction pressure.

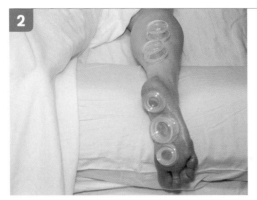

2 Place the second cup directly above the first cup, progressing up the center of the calf toward the knee.

Safety Point

Do not place cups directly over any varicose veins.

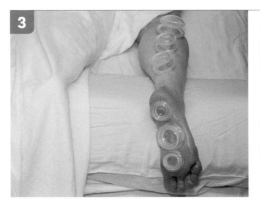

3 Continue placing cups along the back of the calf, progressing up toward the knee. This line of application should be applied straight up the midline. However, if tightness is present more along the outside of the leg, place cups there. For proper assessment, be sure to feel the calf muscles with the fingers to determine areas of tightness before you begin the application. (In this example, the person's leg was much tighter up the outer line of the leg.) The last cup should be well below the soft space behind the knee; this is the popliteal fossa. (See "Endangerment Sites," page 92, for more information.)

To find the end location, place one hand lightly over the back of the knee. Your hand should be completely covering all the soft tissue behind the knee joint. Now slide the hand down toward the ankle approximately 2 fingers' width. The topmost part of the cup should not pass the bottom line of protection created with your hand.

Allow cups to remain in place for a maximum of 3 minutes but no less than a minimum of 30 seconds. Remove cups one at a time, in the order they were applied (from bottom of foot up the calf) for the best relief.

RECOMMENDED AFTER STATIONARY CUPS HAVE BEEN REMOVED: Use either your hand or a cup to lightly encourage recirculation.

EXAMPLE

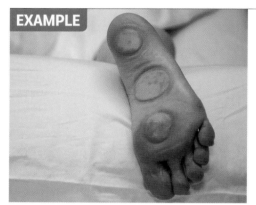

See the stagnation in this case? The lighter coloring suggests a lack of circulation, while the darker color implies a stagnation of blood circulation. Ultimately, this shows that there is some congestion here.

This person has a Morton's neuroma (thickened nerve tissue), just below the toes in the ball of the foot and mild plantar fasciitis. The person reported her foot feeling much better after cups were used.

SELF-CARE APPLICATIONS

It may require some flexibility to work on your own foot. The silicone cups work best here, too — they're easy to manipulate and can be applied with one hand. Notice the positioning of the other hand to hold the foot in place.

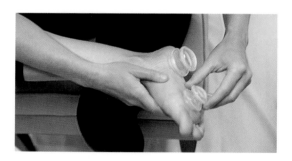

ABDOMINAL APPLICATIONS

The abdominal region is the epicenter of the human body. The visceral organs are contained here, and the musculature in this region (front and back) are crucial for maintaining postural health. The dermis in this region is thinner than that of the back, so any therapeutic cupping applied here should be done with control and consideration to the recipient's comfort and sensitivities. Furthermore, due to this region's delicate internal organs, there should be no vigorous applications. When working in this region, consider any potential contraindications or conditions beyond anatomy where extreme caution is required, including:

- Pregnancy (no abdominal cupping ever)
- Gastric bypass (work with extreme caution, if at all)
- Diastasis recti (separation of abdominal muscles along the midline/linea alba; work with extreme caution over this area if diastasis recti exists, and if the separation is greater than 1.5 inches [3.81 cm] avoid using cups over this area completely)
- Hernias (any hernia other than a basic hiatal hernia, like inguinal epigastric, or incisional hernias)
- Any sections of anatomy that may have been removed (e.g., bowel resections)
- Abdominal meshing (surgically implanted mesh netting, meant to stabilize the abdominal cavity and its contents); work with extreme caution, if at all
- Active flare-up periods associated with irritable bowel syndrome, Crohn's disease and colitis

These are only a few of the contraindications or considerations for when cupping should not be applied in this area. One of the best ways to know if cups can be used in the abdomen is to check with the person's doctor to see if this patient can receive therapeutic abdominal massage or manipulation. If not, then cupping is not recommended in this region.

The most common conditions that benefit from therapeutic cupping — constipation and acid reflux — are addressed in the following pages.

BEFORE YOU START: No cupping or abdominal work should be done for approximately 1 hour after eating so as not to interrupt natural digestion processes.

Constipation

Constipation is a condition that affects many, many people. Defecation is a crucial bodily function and the vast majority of the population experiences irregularity at some time or another. The large intestine, or colon, is an organ at the end of the digestive system's alimentary canal, where it provides the exit point for solid waste from the human body. Optimal functioning of this organ is imperative for good health. The large intestine possesses its own muscle contraction-like movement, called peristalsis, which helps moves waste through this organ. This smooth muscle activity can be easily inhibited, which can create systemic backup and, ultimately, constipation.

Causes

Contributing factors vary widely, but common ones include dehydration, poor nutrition, medications and lack of exercise, to name a few.

Symptoms

Infrequent or irregular bowel movements are the most common symptoms, possibly accompanied by cramping or nausea. Regular bowel movements can vary — from 3 times a day to at least 3 times a week is considered regular. Anything less is classified as constipation.

Cupping and Constipation

The abdomen can be sensitive if someone is constipated. Many people are guarded about abdominal massage for one reason or another, including the fact that it is a personal comfort zone, but cups used here can be quite a welcome experience. Cups lift the tissue to manipulate it, rather than pressing into this protected environment. Plus, if someone is constipated, chances are that the abdominal area already feels tight, so pressing on it for abdominal massage can be uncomfortable. Lifting applied cups in a slow, rhythmic manner as you follow the organ around can mimic its natural peristalsis-like contractions; envision "plucking" the large intestine as you work along its path, loosening whatever may be stuck within the pockets (the huastra).

Following the proper (anatomical) direction of the large intestine — which is clockwise (see detailed directions, page 180) — is imperative. Keep the picture of a clock in mind as you follow the instructions.

Techniques

When applying cups, note the appropriate usage time. Daily applications are not recommended, as this can cause diarrhea. Instead, try applying cups every 2 or 3 days (every 48 to 72 hours) until bowel movements are regular. Occasional applications can also be effective.

Conditions that may also benefit from these applications:

- Inflammatory bowel conditions (e.g., colitis, irritable bowel syndrome). Be sure to treat when not in an active flare-up.
- Indigestion.

Professional Note

The directions on the opposite page are for general applications for constipation. Advanced training with abdominal massage and other therapies may also be used at one's professional discretion.

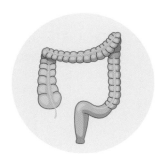

COLON

THE LIFT-AND-RELEASE TECHNIQUE is effective for initial applications. Be sure to lift the cup every time you make a connection; this will further enhance the internal effects.

MOVING CUPS can be very beneficial and soothing here, too. Be sure to lift and release — the Morse Code of Cups (see page 110) — wherever the cup may stick while working through this moving application, especially when addressing the transverse colon, the middle part of the large intestine that passes across the linea alba (band of connective tissue along the midline of the abdomen). If cups "stick," there may be a restriction in the colon (or abdominal tissue) and movement should not be forced.

STATIONARY CUPS are not recommended here, as the intent is to move things along.

More About Techniques

Working in the abdomen should be less about the suction strength and more about the lift and controlled manipulation of the cup. Manual cups are used to demonstrate the Primary Application, while silicone cups are used to demonstrate the Self-Care Application. If choosing to work with manual cups, just be sure to use lighter suction and greater control when using the manual pump gun because one full "pump" of the gun's handle can be stronger than intended. See Chapter 6 for suggestions on optimal usage of equipment. When applying the lift-and-release technique:

- Begin with a lighter suction; as the tissue softens, you may increase the suction pressure if desired. Suction pressure should never be more than a comfortable medium pressure.
- Attach the cup lightly, then gently lift it away from the abdomen until you feel a slight tension engage.
- Slide the cup along the length of the colon, progressing section by section.

Suggestions for making this application most comfortable and effective:

- Be sure to gently lift the cup away from the abdomen every time you apply it. Don't just get suction on the skin and release it. It is this carefully emphasized lift that offers the best results.
- If moving the cup gets stuck, use a lift-and-release technique in that exact location and keep working it along the entire length of the colon. Don't just stop and return to the beginning point again, as a blockage could be causing the cup to stick.

Note

A cup will most likely stick directly in the center of the abdomen as you work across the transverse colon. This is to be expected because the linea alba is located in the midline of the abdomen. (See "Endangerment Sites," page 92, for more information.)

Primary Application

TARGET AREA INCLUDES: The entire length of the large intestine.

Around the Colon

When working to address the large intestine, you must work in logical order. It is important to clear the last sections of the colon before you bring any more material toward this final location. If you started cupping at the beginning of the colon, you could potentially create more rather than less congestion within the organ. Therefore, the rectum area must be cleared, then the descending and sigmoid colon, next the transverse colon, and finally the ascending colon, progressing backwards through each section of the colon. Work the cup in a clockwise direction, moving toward the final exit point with every pass.

The speed of application should also be slower and comfortable, as to mimic the natural smooth muscle contractions of peristalsis through the colon — no fast or aggressive movements when doing this work. Repeat each sequence for a maximum of 3 times but no less than a minimum of 2 times, ending at the 6 o'clock mark with every line of movement.

LIFT-AND-RELEASE OR MOVING CUPS, SUPINE POSITION

BEFORE YOU GET STARTED: Make sure the person is lying comfortably on their back, with a pillow or cushion under their knees to keep legs slightly bent; this allows the abdominal muscles to fully relax. Also, apply lubricant liberally to the entire abdomen to ease appropriate suction pressure and cup movement.

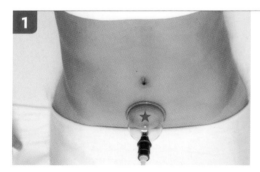

The starting point of this application is over the rectum, the last section of colon before the anus. It is located directly under the belly button and in the middle of the two front hip bones (anterior superior iliac spine, or ASIS). Beginning closest to this exit point will stimulate the clearing process, thereby preparing for the release of all waste that will follow. This location will also be the endpoint for the duration of the treatment.

To locate the starting point (and inevitably the endpoint), first use the fingers to mark a straight line from one hip bone (ASIS) to the other, across the lower abdominal region.

Next, place fingertips at the belly button. Walk them straight down a very short distance, approximately 3 or 4 fingers' width, depending on the size of the abdomen, and stop where the two lines intersect. This should be directly below the belly button and in between the hip bones, at the 6 o'clock mark.

This is the location to begin applying the cup.

Use the lift-and-release technique for a maximum of 5 times but no less than a minimum of 3 times to encourage regional loosening before you begin addressing the rest of the colon.

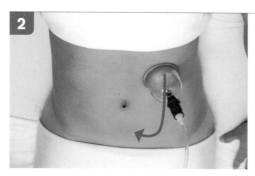

2

Next, address the descending colon, working from top to bottom.

To locate the starting point, draw a straight line from the lower left hip bone up to the underside of left rib cage, approximately one hand's width distance. This middle point along the underside of the front of the left rib cage is where you will begin treating the descending colon.

Lightly attach the cup, lift and slowly move it straight down toward the left hip bone.

Once the cup nears the left hip bone, turn it in toward the midline and finish where you started in Step 1, directly below the belly button (addressing the sigmoid colon into the rectum colon area).

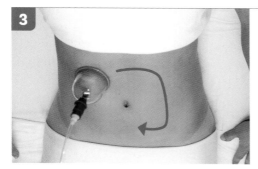

3

Next, address the transverse colon, from the person's right to left across the abdomen.

To locate the starting point, mark a straight line from the right hip bone up to the underside of right rib cage, approximately one hand's width distance. This middle point along the underside of the front of the right rib cage is where you will begin treating the transverse colon.

Lightly attach the cup, lift and slowly move it straight across the abdomen to the junction of the descending colon (Step 2). Note that the linea alba may be tight as you cross over it in the midline.

Then, turn the cup and move it straight down toward the hip bone, addressing the descending colon again (Step 2).

Once the cup nears the left hip bone, turn it in toward the midline and finish where you started in Step 1 (addressing the sigmoid colon into the rectum colon area).

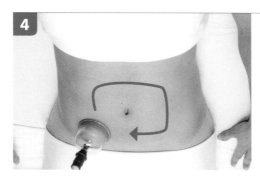

4

Last, address the ascending colon, from bottom to top.

To locate the starting point, place the fingers on the right front hip bone. Place the cup just above the right hip bone, this is the starting point to address the ascending colon.

Next, mark a straight line from the lower right hip bone up to the middle of the underside of the right rib cage (beginning of transverse colon, Step 3). This line up to the middle of the underside of right rib cage is the line of movement to address the ascending colon.

Lightly attach the cup at the lower right hip bone, lift and slowly move the cup straight up toward the middle of the right rib cage.

Then, turn the cup toward the midline and move the cup across the abdomen, addressing the transverse colon again (Step 3).

Next, turn the cup and travel straight down toward the left hip bone, addressing the descending colon again (Step 2).

Once the cup nears the left hip bone, turn it in toward the midline and finish where you started Step 1 (addressing the sigmoid colon into the rectum colon area).

SELF-CARE APPLICATION

When applying these steps, try to use the right hand to address the right side of the abdomen (ascending and parts of the transverse colon) and the left hand to address the left side of the abdomen (parts of the transverse, descending and sigmoid colons and rectum). If you reach across the body with your opposite hand, you may engage abdominal muscles (for example, the oblique muscles cause torso rotation) and cupping will not be as effective. Do the best you can.

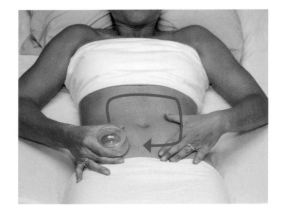

Lying down, face up (supine), is the best position to do this self-care application, whether using the lift-and-release technique or moving cups. Knees should be slightly bent to fully relax the abdominal muscles; place a pillow or cushion behind your knees.

1. Do *not* lift your head up to look for the location, since this will engage the abdominal muscles and the work will not be effective. You can place a pillow under your head for comfort and ease if you require visual assistance.
2. Use one hand to find the locations and the other hand to apply the cup.
3. Follow the detailed instructions in Primary Applications — step-by-step movements to treat your own abdomen for constipation.
4. Try to use your left hand to address the left side of the abdomen (Steps 1, 2 & 3), and your right hand to address the right side of the abdomen (Step 4). The intent is to not engage the abdominal muscles as you work; do the best you can.
5. Repeat this sequence for a maximum of 3 times but no less than a minimum of 2 times, ending at the same 6 o'clock point every time.

Acid Reflux

Acid reflux is a condition that affects many people and generally involves a dysfunction of the cardiac sphincter. Also known as the gastroesophageal sphincter, this valve-like ring of tonic muscle (see Anatomy FYI, below) connects the esophagus to the stomach. When operating correctly, this sphincter relaxes its tonic contraction to allow food materials to enter the stomach, then contracts to close and help contain the stomach's acidic contents. When this process does not function properly, acid reflux occurs. GERD (gastroesophageal reflux disease) is the term associated with chronic, repetitive occurrences of acid reflux, usually more than once a week.

Causes

Acid reflux can be caused by certain food or beverage irritants (spicy foods or high-acid beverages like coffee), smoking, lack of exercise, and pregnancy.

A hiatal hernia can also lead to gastroesophageal acid reflux disease — pressure changes in the abdomen can lead to parts of the stomach passing through the phrenoesophageal membrane, the dividing line of stomach and esophagus.

The most common causes of this damaging pressure can be lifting something heavy, obesity, pregnancy, regular vomiting, constipation and strained bowel movements. Traumatic injury to the abdomen can also cause a hiatal hernia. This sphincter region can also weaken over time due to aging. Pressure changes within the abdomen can also be the result of internal organ damage (such as liver failure), just as similar so-called acid reflux pains can be a sign of other organ dysfunctions (for example, gallstones). Therefore, proper diagnosis is absolutely necessary before attempting to work with cups.

Symptoms

The most common symptom is a burning pain in the central lower chest area. Symptoms may also include belching, nausea, difficulty swallowing and bad breath.

A condition that may also benefit from these applications:

- Indigestion

Remember

No cupping or abdominal work should be done for approximately 1 hour after eating.

Anatomy FYI

Tonic muscles are capable of long, sustained contractions with short terms of relaxation, while phasic muscles remain mostly relaxed, with occasional, rhythmic contractions. The sphincters contained within the gastrointestinal tract are tonic muscles. The rhythmic movements of peristalsis within the gastrointestinal tract are controlled by phasic muscle contractions.

Cupping and Acid Reflux

With its negative pressure into the body, gentle cupping offers effective relief for acid reflux. The intent is to encourage the delicate cardiac sphincter to gently stretch open (in the anatomical direction of the stomach), which will improve its overall muscle tone to help retain stomach acids. Regular applications can promote strengthening of the sphincter, as it is a muscle, and cups can promote beneficial stretching reflexes. If working with a hiatal hernia, you are encouraging the stomach organ itself to slide back down through a delicate — and potentially damaged — membrane. Pressure should be light and any tension against the skin as you move cups should be slow and gentle.

Techniques

THE LIFT-AND-RELEASE TECHNIQUE is helpful when introducing this work to the area, especially for initial applications if someone is sensitive or suffering from GERD.

MOVING CUPS work best here. The movement needs to be controlled and short in distance. The stomach organ's direction is down and on the body's left side (see diagram). Movement with cups should be slow, following the natural direction of the organ.

A STATIONARY CUP will offer some relief for acid reflux as it will help release inflammation around this area of irritation. Be sure to work with lift-and-release and the slightly moving cup for a few applications to ensure regional softening and change before applying a stationary cup. Suction pressure should be light.

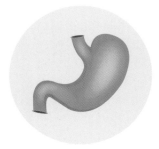

STOMACH

Safety Point

Cupping for acid reflux is absolutely contraindicated during pregnancy. Only non-severe hiatal hernias should be manipulated with cups. One should not attempt to work on any visible protrusions, areas that are painful to touch or severe hernias.

Anatomy FYI

The diaphragm is a large muscle that separates the chest cavity from the abdominal cavity and is the primary muscle involved with breathing.

   The diaphragm can be tight and cause the esophageal hiatus — where the esophagus meets the stomach in the diaphragm — to stretch or tear. Alternatively, the diaphragm can be weak and allow for slack at the sealing junction. Either of these situations can allow for a portion of the stomach organ to slide up into the chest cavity, too.

Primary Application

CARDIAC SPHINCTER FOR ACID REFLUX (MOVING CUP, MINIMAL MOVEMENT)

TARGET AREA INCLUDES: The cardiac, or gastrointestinal, sphincter of the stomach organ.

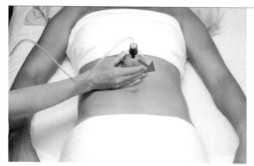

To begin, place the cup directly below the xyphoid process (at the bottom of the sternum), in the upper central region of the abdomen.

To locate the starting point, place the fingertips at the base of the sternum (breastbone). Slowly move the fingers down toward the abdomen until they slip into a soft space at the center of the rib cage, where it meets in the front midline of the body. The xyphoid process is delicate, so do not press hard into this region as you're trying to locate it.

Alternatively, place a medium-sized cup in the center space where the two sides of the rib cage meet. The cup should fit nestled between the ribs and not be placed over the rib cage.

Once the cup fits in this location, begin the application.

Attach the cup lightly, then gently lift the cup away from the abdomen until you feel a slight tension engage.

Maintaining this gentle tension, move the cup very slowly down and to the left, following the natural contour of the stomach. The cup will move a very short distance, the length of your smallest finger maximum.

This small line of movement (down and to the left) may be repeated 3 or 4 times for some relief. You may work this area for a few minutes (recommended to a maximum of 3 minutes, just as with stationary cups). Do not overwork the area.

SELF-CARE APPLICATION

Lying down, face up (supine), is the best position for this application, whether using lift-and-release or a slightly moving cup.

Do not lift your head up to look for the location, since this will engage the abdominal muscles and the work will not be effective. Place a pillow under your head for comfort and ease if you require visual assistance.

1. Use one hand (right) to find the proper location in between the ribs at the upper central abdominal region; see Primary Application for the starting point.
2. Use the other hand to hold and manipulate the cup. It may be easiest to use the left hand to apply the cup, since you'll be moving the cup down and slightly to the left.
3. Attach the cup lightly over the starting point, then gently lift it away from yourself until you feel a slight tension engage.
4. Maintaining this gentle tension, very slowly move the cup down and to your left, following the natural contour of the stomach. The cup will move a very short distance, the length of your smallest finger maximum.

Note

For the greatest and most thoroughly effective application, consider using the full face and head lymphatic drainage application detailed in Chapter 9: "Therapeutic Cupping for Lymphatic Drainage," page 216.

Therapeutic cupping is an effective treatment for the face area. From tension headaches to temporomandibular joint dysfunction (TMJD), applying cups to this delicate region can offer significant relief. In this section, applications are targeted to deal with sinus congestion, TMJD and other tension that may be present in the face. Given that this area is small, it is highly recommended to treat both sides of the face — whether addressing TMJD or sinus congestion — to help maintain overall balance within the region. Adjustments to address other associated discomforts will be made where possible.

Cup Recommendation: Use designated face cupping sets instead of larger body cupping sets in this region. While it may be possible to apply the smallest cup in some full body manual cupping sets, it may still be too big for the anatomical contours of some faces. In addition, even the smallest full body cups are more likely to mark the delicate face tissue.

Example of Face Cupping Sets: Notice the small cup sizes compared to the quarter — perfect for the smaller areas of the face. The smaller squeeze bulbs help regulate suction pressure; it should never be strong enough to mark the delicate face tissue. (Very sensitive tissue may still mark.)

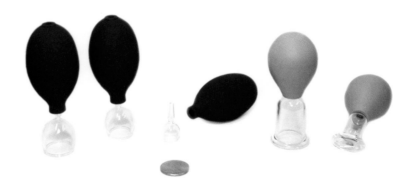

Safety Point

Do not use cupping anywhere cosmetic injections, such as Botox, may have been applied for at least 30 days after they have been administered. Although various cosmetic products vary in how long they may take before tissue can be safely manipulated, the general rule is 30 days. Cupping could dislodge this material from its intended location, moving it to other areas or into circulation. After 30 days, apply only minimal, light cupping over the area if desired.

Temporomandibular Joint Dysfunction (TMJD)

Temporomandibular joint dysfunction, often referred to TMJD, is associated with jaw pain. The temporomandibular joint is formed by the articulation of the temporal bone and the mandible bone (jaw bone), and includes many small, often-fatigued structures like the temporal (located just above the ear, in the hair), masseter and pterygoid muscles (located in the cheek region) as well as tendons, ligaments, synovial membranes, joint capsule and *retrodiscal* tissue (highly vascular structure that contains many nerves).

Causes

Pain in the temporomandibular joint (TMJ) region can be caused by chronic grinding of teeth, clenching of the jaw, dental or orthodontic procedures (such as braces), traumatic injury to the face or jaw, osteoarthritis or other rheumatic disorders that may affect the jaw.

Symptoms

The pain in this area can be described as dull and aching or sharp and piercing. Pain can lead to difficulty opening or closing the mouth, chewing foods or speaking. TMJD can cause a popping or clicking of the jaw or various headaches (tension, cluster, migraines). Pain can be felt in the face, ears, head or neck.

Cupping and TMJD

Cupping is an effective treatment for this tight area. A lot of pressure may already be present in the small region of the cheek, so gentle applications of cupping directly to the jaw muscles can help to hydrate, lift and stretch these small, tight structures. An overall feeling of "openness" can occur quickly.

Techniques

THE LIFT-AND-RELEASE TECHNIQUE is beneficial for initial or regular application. Cupping on the face is quick and effective every time.

MOVING CUPS can be used gently to slide down the masseter muscle (close to the ear, from the cheek bone straight down to the jawline).

STATIONARY CUPS are generally not recommended on the face (some exceptions). The tissue can mark easily, and cups will most likely fall off due to the anatomical structures of the jaw region.

Also, consider applications for neck and shoulder tension (see page 138) to address other muscles often involved in TMJD.

Note

Hair can obstruct the attachment of cups. The more hair, the less a cup will attach. While the bulk of the temporal muscle is located above the ears within the natural hairline, some portions are accessible along the side of the face. If you cannot find a safe and hairless location to attach cup here do not force it, rather massage the location with fingertips instead. Most people do not welcome a lot of oil or lotion to try to make a cup attach here. Bald clients are an exception.

Primary Application

FOR TMJD (BOTH SIDES OF THE JAW)
FACE CUPS: LIFT-AND-RELEASE OR STATIONARY CUP (WHILE MAINTAINING GRIP OF CUP) (SELF-CARE DEMONSTRATED)

TARGET AREA INCLUDES: The temporomandibular joint and masseter and pterygoid muscles.

Using specific face cups allows for more detailed applications, as well as regulated suction pressure control.

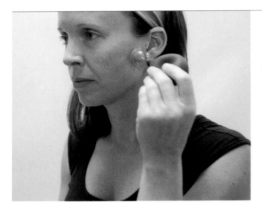

Apply the cup directly over the TMJ jaw area. To locate it, place the fingertips on the highest point of the cheekbone, just in front of the ear. Gently clench the jaw. If applying to someone else, ask them to gently clench their jaw so you can feel the muscles engage. Muscles will "pop" under the fingertips; this is the location to place the cup.
Attach the cup lightly, then gently lift it away from the cheek until you feel a slight tension engage.

OPTION 1: Lift-and-release technique can be applied here repeatedly; repeat this technique in the same exact location, directly over the jaw muscles for quick, effective relief.

OPTION 2: With the regulated suction produced by this squeeze bulb, gentle stationary cups can be applied here. Do not release the grip on the bulb because the cup may fall off the face. Instead, maintain the suction and just hold it in place for a maximum of 30 seconds but no less than a minimum of 10 seconds.
  Whatever method of application you choose, it is recommended to repeat it 3 or 4 times for some relief. However, if it feels really good, then you may work this area for a few minutes (recommended to a maximum of 2 minutes). Do not overwork the area.
  Be sure to treat both sides of the jaw. If not, the jaw may feel uneven. Treating only one side of such a small, tight area can potentially create tension due to compensation.

Anatomy FYI

To locate the *temporal muscle*, gently place your fingertips above an ear and then lightly clench your jaw; you will feel the muscle engage under the fingertips. Try to locate an accessible point that does not involve the temporal artery if you are trying to use cups here.

Optional Application

FACE CUPS: MOVING CUP

The starting location is at the highest point of cheek bone, just in front of the ear (see Primary Application to find this starting point).

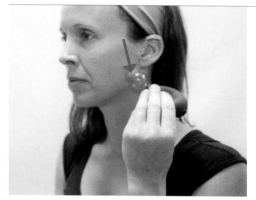
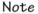

Attach the cup lightly, then gently lift it away from the cheek until you feel a slight tension engage.

Slide the cup down the side of the jaw, from the noted starting location on the cheek bone to the bottom of the jawline.

Be sure to treat both sides of the jaw.

This line of movement may be repeated 3 or 4 times for some relief. If it feels very good, you may work this area for a few minutes (recommended to a maximum of 3 minutes, just as with the stationary cups). Do not overwork the area.

Note

The smallest silicone cup is used for the demonstration. While specified face cups are preferable, using silicone (or the manual pump gun) are available options. You will notice how easily face tissue can mark, however, so control of suction is very important if choosing to work with either of these cupping sets.

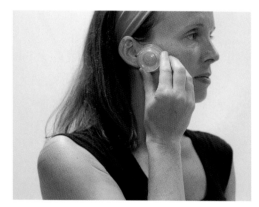

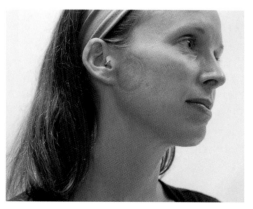

Note

The cheek can be marked very easily if you are not using a face cupping set. BE AWARE.

Sinus Congestion

The face and head can encounter congestion like any other region of the body, especially in the paranasal sinus region, commonly called the sinuses. The sinuses are air-filled cavities that are part of the respiratory system, and these cavities are lined with membranes that create mucus to help contain and remove invasive materials. When this activity is excessively stimulated, such as with seasonal allergies, sinus congestion occurs.

Causes

Sinus congestion — whether as a result of seasonal allergies, the common cold or something more complex, such as sinus polyps — tends to be a common nuisance.

Symptoms

Sinus congestion is accompanied by symptoms like a stuffy nose, headache, the head feeling heavy and an inability to breathe through the nose.

Cupping and Sinus Congestion

Cups gently applied to the face for decongestion provide effective relief without discomfort. This work should be done only with the lightest of suctions. Specific sets of cups designated for just this work — face cups — have very small cups as well as regulated maximum suction control.

Techniques

LIFT-AND-RELEASE APPLICATIONS offer the best quick relief for sinus decongestion, like a massage with your fingertips. This method can be applied at the sides of the nose or just above the eyebrows for sinus decongestion.

STATIONARY CUPS can be challenging to adhere to the surface of a forehead, with its flat edges and bony ridges, so use caution not to press cups too hard against the skin. Do not attempt if it's too frustrating.

MOVING CUPS should be applied for the full head lymphatic drainage application only. Attempting a quick clearing slide next to the nose could potentially back up an otherwise blocked area. Tension or a lymphatic blockage on the side of face or along the base of the jawline (submandibular region), for example, could be causing sinus congestion. See "Face and Head Lymphatic Drainage" in Chapter 9, page 216, for more information.

Note

For best results, follow instructions for the full face and head lymph drainage application (see Chapter 9: "Therapeutic Cupping for Lymphatic Drainage" for more information).

While a full face and head lymphatic drainage application will yield the greatest results, this quick-fix application will still offer some good relief. The small cups create a sense of openness in the areas of major congestion. Naturally, we all tend to massage these points with our fingers for the same reason. It helps stimulate lymph movement in the area as well as relieve sinus pressure when applying cups over these sinus pressure points.

Primary Application

SINUS RELIEF IN TWO LOCATIONS (FACE CUPS: LIFT-AND-RELEASE TECHNIQUE)

Using specific face cups allows for more detailed applications, as well as regulated suction pressure control.

TARGET AREA INCLUDES: Face points for sinus relief.

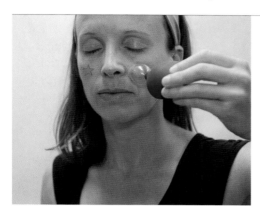

FIRST LOCATION: Apply the cup just to the side of the nostril (first one side, then the other). To locate this point, place the index fingertip directly beside the outside of the nostril. Move the finger slowly over in the direction of the ear, approximately 1 finger's width, where you will bump into some bone; this is the start of the zygomatic arch cheek bone. Place the cup just to the inside of this bony location, next to the nostril; instinctually, we may rub this area with our fingers when sinuses are congested.

Attach the cup lightly, then gently lift the cup away from the face until you feel a slight tension engage.

Use this method of application to apply the lift-and-release technique 3 or 4 times in the same location.

Repeat on the other side.

Use the lightest suction pressure; the technique is less about the suction and more about the *lift of the cup* once it is attached to the skin to create space. This gentle technique offers subtle decompression of the congested sinus area.

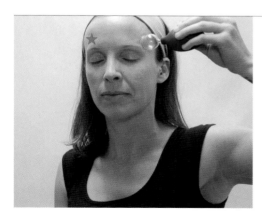

SECOND LOCATION: Apply the cup just above the eyebrow line (first one side, then the other). To locate this point, place the fingertips on the eyebrow. Slide the fingers up a very short distance to find a flat surface of forehead, just above the orbital ridge (bony ridges over the eye). Place the cup just above the eyebrow on the available flat surface of the forehead; instinctually, we rub here with our fingers when sinuses are congested.

Attach the cup lightly, then gently lift the cup away from the face until you feel a slight tension engage.

Use this method of application to apply the lift-and-release technique 3 or 4 times across the top of the eyebrow, working from the center to the outside edge of the eyebrow. Repeat on the other side.

Use the lightest suction pressure; the technique is less about the suction and more about the *lift of the cup* once it is attached to the skin.

CHAPTER 9

Therapeutic Cupping for Lymphatic Drainage

While a full body application will be demonstrated in this chapter, you will also learn how to apply cups in specific regions of the body. A full body application is not necessary to treat a swollen ankle, for example, but you will want to apply these draining movements to the person's entire leg. Chapter 8 also references lymphatic applications to encourage the movement or recirculation of lymph after specific applications. Here's a recap of terms first used in Chapter 8 to more accurately locate areas of the body for the application of cups:

- **Proximal** means *closer* to the torso.
- **Distal** means *further* from the torso.
- **Lateral** means more to the *outside* or away from the midline of the body.
- **Medial** means more to the *inside* or closer to the midline of the body.

HOW THE LYMPHATIC SYSTEM WORKS

One of the most profound effects of therapeutic cupping takes place within the lymphatic system. As part of the circulatory system, the lymphatic system is responsible for removing waste from the body, as well as fighting off infections and distributing certain nutrients from the digestive tract into the bloodstream. Therapeutic cupping not only draws out interstitial debris from within the layers of soft tissue, bringing it up to the surface for lymphatic disposal, but it also has the ability to support the movement of lymph fluids along their natural drainage pathways, leading to an overall improved sense of well-being.

Basics of Lymphatic System Anatomy

The lymphatic system collects, filters and disposes of as much metabolic waste as possible. All the cellular debris (cellular waste, old blood, medications) found within the interstitial fluid enters the lymphatic system through flap valves in the lymph capillaries, then travels through progressively larger lymph vessels toward ultimate removal through the main drainage ducts in the upper torso (right and left thoracic ducts). The system flows in one direction, from distal regions of the body (near the skin's surface, and from the furthest points, like the hands and feet) toward the heart. Unlike the cardiovascular system, however, where the heart pumps fluids around the body, the lymphatic system relies on muscle movement, the valves in lymph vessels and the negative pressure in the chest when we breathe to move lymph along its route. (See Chapter 3: "Therapeutic Benefits on the Body Systems" for more information.)

Lymphatics 101

Lymph in the more superficial layers has no specific direction, which can easily result in misguided lymph fluids. Therefore, various methods of lighter-pressured manual therapies are used to move lymph along its natural drainage pathways to support the system's vital health processes.

How Does Lymph Become Stagnant?

The lymphatic system can become challenged by any number of contributing factors, including sedentary lifestyles, tight muscles, injuries, repetitive motions, surgeries, medications, environmental exposures and pathogenic substances (such as chemical fumes or second-hand smoke). Lymphatic stagnation is a fairly common issue of varying proportions. Just as interstitial debris can cause a sort of systemic backup within the body (see page 22 for a definition of "interstitial debris"), so too can any general stagnation of lymph. Compounding the problem, the body has the ability to retain residue from any such stagnation for months and even years.

If inflammation was present in the body at some time, either due to injuries, illnesses, surgeries, toxicity or systemic conditions, the lymphatic system can become challenged. Here's how this happens: Inflammation can occur in the body for many reasons and to varying degrees (acute versus chronic). Inflammation can literally "cook" and dehydrate soft tissues, which directly affects all the interstitial fluids, too. Just as heat changes the integrity of soft tissues, so too does it alter the composition of lymph fluids, causing them to thicken and hindering their natural passage through needed areas. This results in the stagnation of displaced waste fluids, a sort of ripple effect of backup in the body.

THERAPEUTIC THOUGHT: SURFACE COLORS

During my years of practice, I have witnessed cupping bring up many old stagnations to the surface. A few examples are dark purple marks reminiscent of injuries from many years ago on one individual, gray colors on someone who hasn't smoked cigarettes for more than 15 years, and even yellow colors and a taste of medication in an adult who was treated with these medications for an ailment during her youth.

Retention of any inflammation can also hinder the body's natural healing mechanisms. Wherever inflammation occurs (for example, an injury), the pH level of the site shifts, becoming more acidic to initiate the inflammatory healing processes. While this process is finishing its work, the body tries to rid the area of the acidic waste materials to allow healthy oxygen to return to the site. When the area is too restricted, however, or the body is not allowed to fully recover, such as exercising before a sports injury is fully recovered, this alkaline-regulating action cannot be fully completed and the area can remain in a more acidic state, never fully returning to a healthy condition.

The term *pH* (the potential of hydrogen) is used for the ratio of acid to alkalinity in any liquid. In the human body, the pH ranges from 0 to 14; the lower the number, the higher the acidity. Body chemistry functions best at a high-oxygen, low-acid state. An excess of oxygen is called *hyperoxia* and can occur from breathing oxygen at higher than normal atmospheric pressure. In dysfunction or disease, the body can be in a high-acid, low-oxygen state, known as *hypoxia*.

How Cupping Benefits Overall Lymphatic System Functions

Cups facilitate not only the vacuum-like lymphatic clearing of localized underlying tissues (as shown in Chapter 8), but also enhance the natural drainage process — a systemic "flushing" of various residues and waste materials (such as lactic acid, heat, old blood). Using the lighter applications discussed in this chapter, cups will address the more superficial layers of anatomy, where lymph filtration occurs, with negative pressure. The subtle lifting action of lighter cupping encourages a gentle opening of the flap valves that are part of the intermediate lymphatic drainage pathways. These valves can also become challenged when lymph fluids are too thick and limit or hinder lymph movement, potentially resulting in edema (see sidebar, opposite page). When given directional guidance, cups have an impressive capability of simultaneously moving lymph fluids along their natural routes.

- The lift-and-release technique mimics the natural, rhythmic opening of the flap valves along their routes.
- Slow and gentle moving cups offer a soothing, wave-like motion along the same pathways.
- Wherever you move the cup, fluid will follow.

All along the path of application, cups offer lifting release and openness to any previously obstructed areas of drainage (tight muscles, scar tissue), ultimately resulting in improved circulation.

While more complicated edema-related conditions should be referred to a manual lymph drainage specialist, using cups in this fashion can offer some benefits. Whether applying cups for chronic edema conditions (such as repetitive sports injuries or chronic inflammatory conditions) or as a detoxifying treatment, this style of cupping offers an entirely new dimension of therapeutic benefit to the body.

What is Edema?

Edema is an excess of lymph fluid in interstitial spaces, usually defined as just swelling. The difference is that swelling occurs as a response to inflammation, whereas edema can occur without inflammation; the tissue fluids swell due to some other fluid dysfunction. Edema usually occurs in the legs, ankles and feet, though it can also occur in the arms and throughout the body. Various complicated cases of edema can result from multiple contributing factors, including cardiovascular, kidney or liver diseases; certain pharmaceuticals, such as steroids; hypothyroidism; or certain autoimmune conditions, such as lupus.

Some of the most common compromised edema conditions include:

- **Acute or new edema** is usually caused by injury (a sprained ankle), surgery (such as mastectomy surgery, where lymph nodes have been removed in the axilla) or problems with all the body systems (toxic overload).
- **Pitting edema** is a form of edema where the skin retains an impression whenever pressure is applied. This indentation will disappear after a short time.
- **Lymphedema** is a disturbance of lymphatic functions, often caused by surgeries such as mastectomies, lymph node surgeries and radiation. While many cases of edema occur in the extremities (arms and legs), some cases of lymphedema can involve the entire body.
- **Lipedema**, or **lipoedema**, is a congenital condition characterized by an excess of adipose tissue in the subcutaneous layers of body tissue, most commonly affecting women.
- **Anasarca** is a term used for generalized swelling throughout the body, usually due to various system failures.
- **Ascites** is an excess of fluids in the abdominal cavity (swollen stomach).

Cupping Treatment

Any form of *autoimmune-related edema* (for example, lupus) can be addressed with cups, as long as the individual is not suffering from an active flare-up (any time too much fluid is being retained).

Any case of *acute edema* should be approached similarly to acute inflammation (see "Working with Inflammation" in Chapter 10) or evaluated for any contraindications (see Chapter 5: "Safe Cupping").

Any form of edema that would be contraindicated for massage or bodywork should not be cupped, but rather referred to a specialist. If you're not sure, do not use cups — safety is most important with any form of therapeutic bodywork, with or without cups.

Anatomy FYI

The lymphatic system is composed of superficial, intermediate and deep drainage structures. The superficial drainage collection starts just below the surface of the skin. Then the system progresses slightly deeper into the body, evolving into the intermediate, flap valve–containing lines of drainage, which exist below the dermis but above the muscles. Still deeper and further along the drainage pathways are the lymph nodes and other drainage and filtration bodies, such as the cisterna chyli (in the upper middle abdominal region), left and right thoracic ducts and spleen.

Helping or Hurting Lymphatic Drainage

Whether the lymphatic system is working to fight infection or to heal injured tissues, this work should not be directly disturbed while it is in a new or acute situation. Be sure the illness has been addressed and the patient is on the mend before attempting to clear the area and interrupt infection-fighting lymph. During a sinus infection, for example, the lymph nodes in the head are working to fight off agents that caused the infection and should be allowed to do their work around the sinuses. Working too early on a patient can inhibit progress; wait *at least* 72 hours from the time of initial sickness before attempting to clear the area. The sicker the person, however, the longer the acute phase may last.

For injured tissue, facilitating lymphatic drainage around or above the area of swelling (closer to the torso if on a limb, or in the direction of drainage if on the torso) can support the overall healing process. During an active or acute inflammation, however, the same guidelines apply: the immediate location should not be directly disturbed. In this injured area, the lymphatic system is working to stabilize, heal and rebuild the damaged tissues. Again, wait *at least* 72 hours before attempting to clear the area, only working proximal to the area when the time is right. The more severe the injury, the longer the acute phase may last. And remember, no cupping directly over sites of *acute inflammation.*

Safety Point

Neither of the two scenarios with acutely inflamed, lymph-concentrated areas described below should receive direct cupping. Any direct cupping would only be harmful, not helpful.

1. If tissue seems too compromised (for example, pitting edema, when you lightly touch the skin and a dent remains), it is highly recommended not to use cupping. Seek professionally trained assistance for such conditions.
2. Anyone who has had lymph nodes removed (such as many breast cancer survivors) do not have normal lymph drainage and can suffer damage if the person applying cups brings fluid to a region where there are no longer lymph nodes, such as the axilla.

Deeper Levels of Lymphatic Drainage

This section will focus on encouraging full body, universal lymphatic drainage applications on a deeper, *intermediate* level, rather than the superficial level. The applications discussed here are unique variations of full body lymphatic drainage, a style of therapeutic cupping that safely addresses layers of tissue on a deeper level that is just below the superficial level. Traditionally, the more superficial drainage pathways are addressed with either hands or high-quality vacuum machines, as true superficial lymphatic drainage therapies cause no hyperemia (redness due to increased blood flow to the area), and working with only the superficial lymphatic system requires an incredible amount of training and control. Since most varieties of cups, even when lightly applied, still penetrate deeply beyond the superficial drainage system, the applications shown here approach this work at the intermediate level.

While one area of the body may be the focus of an application (for example, cellulite reduction in the hips, fluid retention in the legs), the lymphatic system works on a more general scale. This means that if you are choosing to focus on one particular area, such as a swollen ankle, apply cups to the general area for the greatest results. In other words, encourage drainage to the entire extremity, not just the lower leg in the case of a swollen ankle. Similarly, if you are choosing to focus on an area of cellulite, such as the gluteal hip region, address the entire core, which includes the midsection and abdomen.

Who Should Consider Cupping for Lymphatic Drainage?

Consider applications for lymphatic drainage if an individual is

- Experiencing heavy, lethargic or lingering muscle aches that won't go away naturally. Encouraging lymphatic drainage can help jump-start the body's natural methods of detoxification.
- Suffering from repetitive colds or a general feeling of malaise that doesn't seem to go away. While proper medical diagnosis is always recommended to confirm a cold and rule out other possible illnesses, cupping the delicate lymphatic system may help facilitate its natural function of flushing out cellular waste from destroyed infectious materials (viruses).
- Experiencing poor overall circulation. An application of cups can help support the venous return of blood from the extremities and blood circulation.
- Living a sedentary lifestyle. Such lifestyles can inhibit the natural flow of lymph that muscle contractions facilitate. The abdomen can accumulate a lot of congestion with more sedentary lifestyles, as the constant compression on the inguinal lymph nodes (see Anatomy FYI, next page) can inhibit their natural, powerful draining functions.

Anatomy FYI

The *inguinal lymph nodes* are located in the groin area, both above and below your hip bones. They work to drain the entire lower body into your cisterna chyli (located in the upper middle abdominal region), which is connected to the bottom of the thoracic ducts, the main drainage locations for the entire body.

- Accumulating body aches from overexertion, either from exercise or playing or training for a sport, or has suffered a traumatic injury that resulted in inflammation. Inflammation can dry out bodily tissues, altering the layers of anatomy where lymph vessels travel and thereby inhibiting optimal lymphatic drainage. Cupping can help express waste (inflammation, lactic acid) from muscles into the lymphatic system while simultaneously replenishing previously dehydrated tissues with oxygen-rich blood supplies. Out with the waste stagnations, in with healthy blood.
- Undergoing surgery or has acquired scars from surgery. Any surgical procedure that makes an incision into the body is essentially cutting through the web of delicate lymph vessels that runs through the body.
- Taking medications for a prolonged period, such as steroids. Years of medications can hinder natural removal of lymph because such substances can cause lymph to thicken and potentially overload the system with toxicity. Drug addictions can take a similar toll; in fact, the longer the drug use, the more challenged the lymphatic system. Cupping can help to gently clear the system.

When to Use Lymphatic Cupping: A Few Examples

Cellulite: While there may be unpleasant "dimples" isolated to the gluteal and hip regions, don't stop short by focusing only on these regions. Because the hips are part of the midsection of the body, a full body application or, at the very least, cupping in the general region (the abdomen, torso and upper legs) will bring the greatest benefit.

Swollen ankles: If poor circulation is to blame for localized swelling, the entire body could benefit from stimulated lymphatic movement. While you may choose to focus only on the legs, remember that the lymphatic system is a unit and will yield greater results if addressed in its entirety. If you must focus only on swollen ankles, at least address the lower abdominal region so the inguinal (upper and lower) lymph nodes are stimulated, thereby moving this lymph fluid toward the cisterna chyli and into the thoracic ducts.

Scar tissue: Whether scar tissue is from a cut to the skin (surgery) or is formed from repetitive injuries (sprinting leg muscles), lymph cannot pass through this obstructive tissue. Following the drainage pathways *through* whatever body part the scar tissue is involved with will help to restore natural, unobstructed drainage to the tissues located in the area.

GUIDELINES FOR THERAPEUTIC CUPPING FOR LYMPHATIC DRAINAGE

1. **Pressure should be lighter.** Attempts to move lymph fluid should be gentle; lighter suction pressure will more effectively address surface layers of tissue where lymph drainage passes through.

2. **Use moving cups or lift-and-release techniques — no stationary cups.** The intention with lymphatic drainage is to move fluid, not create areas of stagnation that using stationary cups might promote. Moving cups can create a wonderful "wave" or movements of fluid as the cups slide along the drainage pathways. Furthermore, the lift-and-release technique is effective for mimicking the true flap valve–like lifting mechanism of the lymphatic vessels. Use either of these techniques to address the tissue accordingly, or combine the two as you deem necessary (known as the Morse Code of Cups — see page 110).

3. **Cup used should be larger in size.** When attempting lymphatic drainage, you are working to clear lymph in the entire area being treated. Your intention here is not to focus on any one spot, so a small cup on the back isn't as effective as a larger cup. Yes, your ankle will require a smaller cup than your back, but relative to the body part you are working on, be sure to work in a broader application with cup sizes.

4. **Movements should be slow, rhythmic, repetitive.** The movement of cups along the drainage pathways should be slower and smoother than with any other deeper cupping work. Think of the movements as long, draining strokes to encourage fluid to move along its way — nothing too vigorous or aggressive. You should also pass over the same body line with the cup a few times. Just as massage strokes are multiple in their passes, so should the technique be with cups. Consider making three to five passes over the line of movement in each body section for a universal, detoxifying treatment.

5. **Treat and drain more proximal or central regions before attempting distal areas.** If you are attempting to move fluid from an ankle, for example, be sure to address the thigh first, then the lower leg. If there is anything imposing upon the lymphatic system along the drainage route, this method of treatment is necessary for optimal effect. In the case of a swollen ankle, perhaps there is something in the groin or thigh that is causing fluid to become stagnant and pool at the ankle. Draining an entire limb in logical order yields the greatest results with the least amount of harm. Imagine a clogged shower drain: you must address what is clogging the drain before expecting the standing water to drain. If you start draining the ankle at its most distal location, you may cause more damage or backup.

6. **Be aware of the drainage direction.** On the opposite page is a basic map of the intermediate level for lymph drainage pathways and the direction in which they should be worked. Be sure to follow the map to the best of your ability. If you are unfamiliar with the lymphatic pathways or have any questions, be sure to contact a manual lymphatic drainage therapist for treatment or do more research before you begin.

7. **When in doubt, refer out.** While the directions may look simple, there may be cause for pause or question. There are countless reasons why someone *should not receive cups from an untrained bodyworker.* Such is the case with patients who are post-surgery for cancer (such as mastectomy) and don't have lymph nodes in their axilla region. The same goes for treating an individual with lymphedema. These techniques are intended for people who are generally in good health and applied by professional bodyworkers. Those using cups for self-care should follow these guidelines when assessing to treat themselves. There is no shame in referring to a specialist in such cases.

ANTERIOR (LEFT) AND POSTERIOR (RIGHT) INTERMEDIATE LYMPH DRAINAGE PATHWAYS

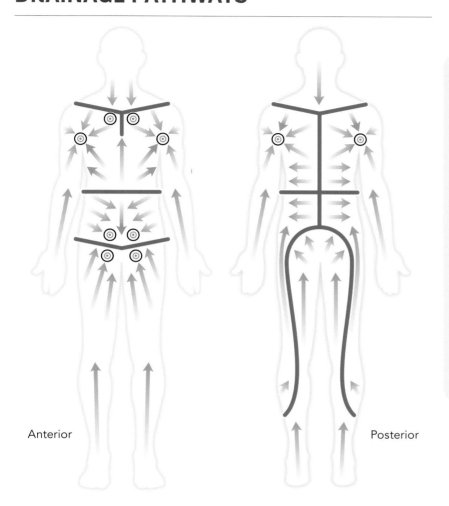

Anterior

Posterior

Safety Point

- Cups should be lighter in suction when addressing lymphatic movement.
- Techniques should be limited to moving or lift-and-release only — no stationary cups.
- Follow the map of intermediate lymphatic drainage pathways if you are unsure of directions in which to move cups.

Before You Begin

Assess the state of the abdominal area, which is the most proximal, central region of the body. If you or the person being treated suffers from excessive abdominal congestion, such as constipation, consider treating the abdominal area first before cupping for full body lymphatic drainage (see Chapter 8 for the suggested application for constipation, page 178). This allows you to "unclog" the body's drain before you begin bringing the lymph material into the abdominal region. It also offers the body a little more support to deal with pre-existing challenges. If you are not sure about excessive abdominal congestion, go ahead and treat this area first (during the same session) and then proceed to address the entire body.

Make sure cups are ready and within reach, along with oil and a hand towel to wipe the oil off your hands.

THERAPEUTIC CUPPING FOR FULL BODY LYMPHATIC DRAINAGE

Note

The instructions contained in this chapter are suggested for a general, universal and overall safe application of therapeutic cupping for detoxifying and general lymph drainage purposes. Specially trained manual lymph drainage therapists may choose to interpret these applications to better suit their training.

CUPPING 101

Remember, switch to the lift-and-release technique for any location where a moving cup is uncomfortable or difficult to use, such as any tight area of tissue, like along the sides of the legs over the IT band. You may choose to mix moving cups and lift-and-release at any time.

Initial applications may prove to be more sensitive, as the body is not familiar with the concept of negative pressure therapies. Opting to incorporate the lift-and-release technique wherever needed will ensure a more comfortable and effective experience.

Duration

When working on the entire body with this style of cupping, the length of time needed to complete such a treatment may vary. On average, the entire body can be treated in 30 minutes to 1 hour. The variation in time can depend on the pace, repetition and lines of movement involved. As suggested in this chapter, limiting the count on each line of movement to no less than 3 but no more than 5 strokes ensures a thoroughly safe and effective, universal application of cups for lymphatic drainage.

If you are following these instructions to address one localized region, however, such as addressing challenges to lower body circulation (for example, chronically swollen ankles) or addressing the entire arm for carpal tunnel treatments, then the length of time will be adjusted accordingly. It might take 5 to 10 minutes to address the arm, 15 to 20 minutes to address the lower body.

Whatever application you choose, cupping should not be repeated daily; rather, allow 48 hours between each session. Waiting this long is necessary to allow the various tissues and drainage vessels involved to completely process the cupping, resettle to their natural state and be ready for any further manipulations, if required. (See "How Often Can Cups Be Used?" on page 28 for more information.)

Direction of Application

When working on the entire body, divide it into two halves — left and right — for each section. You can choose to begin on either side of the body, but I prefer the left side because the thoracic duct, which is located in the left upper chest area, drains most of the body. What is most important is to be methodical and thorough with this treatment.

This chapter includes the directions of application for full body lymphatic drainage with cups. However, if you are choosing to address one particular location of the body (for example, a swollen ankle), be sure to address the entire region and its relationship to the torso with respect to overall lymph drainage pathways. Remember, the lymphatic system functions best when any therapeutic application considers the entire region involved with the drainage process.

The arm, for carpal tunnel syndrome: Begin by opening up the axilla (armpit) region ("unclog the drain"), then address the upper arm and then the lower arm; addressing the most proximal region (the axilla region, then the upper arm) before addressing the more distal region (the lower arm).

The lower body, for circulation challenges (such as chronic edema-induced swollen ankles): Address the abdominal core region, opening up the inguinal (groin) lymph nodes, then address the thigh region (front and back) before addressing the lower leg (front and back); addressing the more proximal regions (abdomen, then thigh) before addressing the more distal region (the lower leg).

The entire midsection, for overall abdominal health and circulation: Begin in the lower abdominal points located between the two front hip points and below the belly button, as instructed to locate in Step 9 on page 210, before beginning the draining movements throughout the abdominal region, starting in the lower region of the abdomen, then progressing up the torso before ending just below the breast tissue; addressing the more proximal region (the inguinal lymph node region) before addressing the more distal (the upper midsection, just below breast tissue).

Recommended Sequence for Full Body Application

- Address the midsection of the body before you work on the limbs, starting with the back of the torso. The entire left half of the torso will be drained to the left side of the body, in a line from the armpit down to the top of the hip (as demonstrated on page 204). Repeat the process on the right side of the torso, draining the entire right half of the torso to the right side of the body, in a line from the armpit down to the top of the hip.
- Next, proceed to the back of the entire left upper arm (as demonstrated on page 204), then repeat the process on the back of the entire right upper arm.
- Proceed to the back of the entire left leg (as demonstrated on page 207: gluteal region and hips, then back of thigh, then lower leg), then repeat the process on the back of the entire right leg.
- In the abdomen, address the left side of the abdomen (from hip bones, progressing up the side of the abdomen, ending just below the breast tissue; see page 210), then repeat the process on the right side.
- Address the front of the entire left leg (as demonstrated on page 212: upper thigh, then lower leg), then repeat the process on the front of the entire right leg.
- Address the entire front of the left arm (as demonstrated on page 214: upper arm, then forearm), then repeat the process on the entire front of the right arm.
- The upper chest region can be drained on the left side first (starting at the midline of the body, below the clavicle but above the breast tissue, then move out toward the armpit), then the right side.

Full Body Cupping Sequence

STEP 1: THE MIDSECTION, BACK OF THE BODY (LEFT SIDE)

Begin by instructing the person to be in the prone position, arms relaxed and extended off the sides of the table (if comfortable). You'll begin by addressing the back of the midsection in the lower back, just above the hip bones (posterior iliac crest).

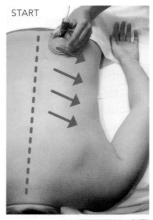
START

- The starting point is along the side of the spine (shown right), just above the hip bones. To locate this point, find the place where the base of the spine meets the top of the iliac crest/back hip bone points; place the cup to the side of the spine and just above the back hip bone.
- Attach the cup lightly, then gently lift it away from the body until you feel a slight tension engage.
- Move the cup from the midline of the body (spine) out to the sides (endpoints). Detach the cup here, then return it to the starting point.
- Repeat each line of movement for a minimum of 3 times but no more than a maximum of 5 times.
- Progress your way up the back, one cup width at a time, ending at the bottommost point of the shoulder blade (about one hand's width from the top of the shoulders). From the front of the body, this is just below the breast tissue.

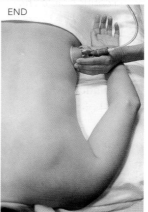
END

Repeat this sequence on the right side of the body.

STEP 2: STIMULATING REGIONAL LYMPH NODES

Before continuing in this area, apply the lift-and-release technique just outside the axilla (armpit), which will stimulate all the lymph nodes located in this region to receive lymph from the surrounding areas. If excessive congestion is present, you may *very lightly* — barely any suction at all — apply the lift-and-release technique 3 to 5 times directly in the armpit.

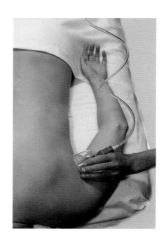

- The starting point is on the posterior border of the axilla.
- To locate this point, place the fingers at the outside of the shoulder blade where the arm joins the torso. Place the cup here, just outside of the actual armpit region, approximately one finger's width.
- Attach the cup, then gently use the lift-and-release technique for a minimum of 3 times but no more than a maximum of 5 times in the same location.

Repeat this sequence on the right side of the body.

STEP 3: THE UPPER BACK

Begin addressing the upper back at the bottom of the shoulders, where Step 1 ended, just below the shoulder blade.

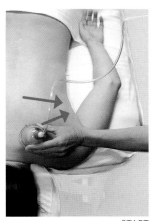
START

- The starting point is along the side of the spine, in line with the bottom of the shoulder blade (shown right).
- Attach the cup lightly, then gently lift it away from the body until you feel a slight tension engage.
- Move the cup from the midline of the body out to the sides, close to the axilla (armpit), where Step 2 was applied. Detach the cup here, then return to the starting point.
- Progress your way around the shoulder blade. One cup width at a time, move the cup in a triangle-like pattern over the entire shoulder blade, working out toward the axilla endpoint every time.

Note

If you cannot slide the cup over the shoulder blade comfortably, use the lift-and-release technique to move across it.

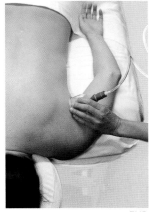
END

- Repeat each line of movement for a minimum of 3 times but no more than a maximum of 5 times.
- End addressing the upper back along the outside of shoulder blade, just before the arm begins.

Repeat this sequence on the right side of the body.

Note

The upper border for this area is along the tops of the shoulders, separate from the upper shoulder drainage area. Naturally, this small region at the top of the shoulders drains forward to the clavicle.

Upper Shoulder Drainage

To locate this separate area, lightly touch the spine around the T1/T2 vertebrae at the base of the neck, where the neck meets the top of the shoulders. Follow a diagonal line out toward the top of shoulder, traveling along the bony ridge of the spine of the scapula; this is the uppermost part of the shoulders, the upper trapezius muscle region. The area *above* this line will be addressed in Step 4.

If you are having difficulty finding this area, take your hands and bring them together on your spine behind the base of your neck. Slowly slide the fingers around the sides of your neck, over the top of your shoulders, coming forward toward the front of your body and ending at your clavicle (collarbones). This space is very short, your hand's width at most.

STEP 4: UPPER SHOULDERS

Begin addressing the upper shoulders near the top of the scapula, just above the area Step 3 addressed, working over top of the shoulder blade.

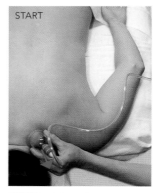
START

▶ The starting point is along the top of the scapula (shoulder blade, shown right). If you are having difficulty finding this location, review how to locate the separate upper shoulder drainage area in Step 3.
▶ Attach the cup lightly, then gently lift it away from the body until you feel a slight tension engage.
▶ Move the cup from the top of the shoulder a short distance (less than one hand's width), around the side of the neck and end just before the clavicle. Detach the cup here, then return to starting point.

Note

A moving cup may be challenging due to the anatomical contour and small space. Use the lift-and-release technique if necessary.

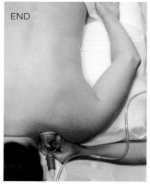
END

▶ Repeat this short line of movement for a minimum of 3 times but no more than a maximum of 5 times.
▶ End addressing the upper shoulders just inside the clavicle.

Repeat this sequence on the right side of the body.

STEP 5: BACK OF THE UPPER ARM

It is recommended to position the arm off the side of the table (shown right). This exposes the triceps area and avoids direct cupping to the inside of the arm, where superficial blood vessels are located.

Begin treating the back of the upper arm (triceps) near the elbow.

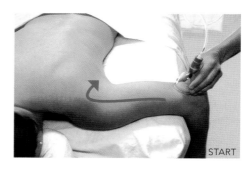
START

▶ The starting point is above the elbow joint, where a larger cup fits comfortably on the back of the arm.
▶ Attach the cup lightly, then gently lift it away from the body until you feel a slight tension engage.
▶ Move the cup in toward the body along the length of the upper arm; turn the cup slightly downward once the arm meets the body and finish along the outer edge of the shoulder blade and just outside the axilla (armpit), where Step 2 was applied. Detach the cup here, then return to the starting point.

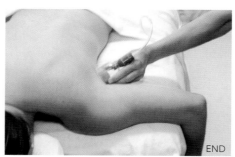
END

▶ Repeat this line of movement for a minimum of 3 times but no more than a maximum of 5 times.
▶ End addressing the back of the upper arm, finishing the back of the upper body.

Repeat this sequence on the right side of the body.
The next area to treat is the leg.

STEP 6: HIPS AND GLUTEAL REGION

Begin addressing the back of the leg at the hip, working one entire leg before the other (shown right).

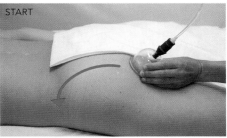

▸ The starting point is at the bottommost aspect of the gluteal cheek region, above the beginning of the back of the thigh, where the leg meets the gluteal region. There is often a "bubble-like bump" where the gluteal region begins; this is where to begin.

▸ Attach the cup lightly, then gently lift it away from the body until you feel a slight tension engage.

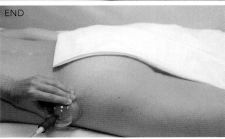

▸ Move the cup up at a slight angle, toward the outside of the hip. This endpoint will be the same as the endpoint in Step 1, where this sequence began, at the outermost aspect of the hip (shown right). Detach the cup here, then return to the starting point.

▸ Repeat each line of movement for a minimum of 3 times but no more than a maximum of 5 times.

Note

Each hip size will vary; cover the area one cup width at a time. In this example, two lines are demonstrated.

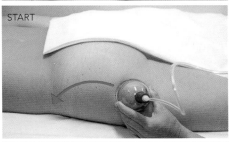

Safety Point

For all leg applications: No cups should be applied directly over varicose veins. Skip over them entirely or avoid any region with excessive vascular damage.

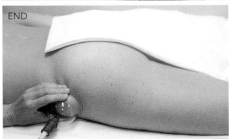

Next, progress to the back of the thigh, same leg.

STEP 7: BACK OF THE THIGH

The back of the thigh should be sectioned in half lengthwise. The outer half will go to the outside of the hip (same endpoint as the first line of movement in Step 1); the inner half will go to the inside.

Begin addressing the back of the thigh just *above* the beginning of the back of the knee endangerment site called the popliteal fossa (see "Endangerment Sites," page 92 for more detailed information). Begin with the outer half of the thigh, then move to the inner half.

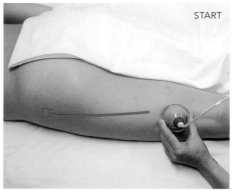

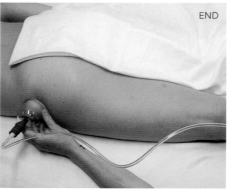

- ▸ The starting point is just above the popliteal fossa, within the hamstring muscles.
- ▸ To locate it, center one hand over the soft space in the back of the knee; this is the popliteal fossa, where many nerves, blood vessels and lymph nodes are located, and cups should not be directly applied here.
- ▸ Attach the cup lightly in the outer half of the hamstring muscles, above the designated endangerment space. Then gently lift it away from the body until you feel a slight tension engage.
- ▸ Move the cup up at a slight angle, toward the outside of the hip — where the first endpoint was for Step 1, just above the lateral hip bone on the side of the body. Detach cup here, then return to the starting point.
- ▸ Repeat each line of movement for a minimum of 3 times but no more than a maximum of 5 times.

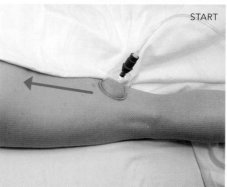

Repeat this sequence on the inner half of the thigh.

The line of movement will be from just above the knee on the inner half of the thigh, ending below the posterior groin area. Larger bodies may require multiple cup widths to address the entire thigh; however, be sure to keep the thigh divided in half lengthwise, for both the applications on the outer and inner thigh.

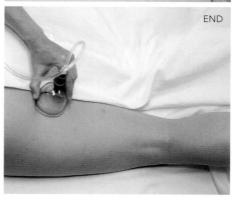

Note

Avoid going all the way up the inner thigh, as this can be a bit personal and the femoral triangle (groin area) will address the fluid appropriately brought into this region. (See Chapter 5: "Safe Cupping" for more information.)

Next, treat the back of the lower leg.

Drainage of Lower Leg Is Optional

This application is not required when doing a basic full body treatment. It may be useful to drain the lower leg if you are already focused on treating the leg for such conditions as plantar fasciitis (heel pain) or fluid retention. Treating the upper thigh will directly benefit lower leg drainage — clearing a proximal area before a distal area has a direct effect on distal lymphatic drainage activity. Step 13 is also optional.

STEP 8: (OPTIONAL) LOWER LEG

Begin treating the back of the lower leg just above the ankle.

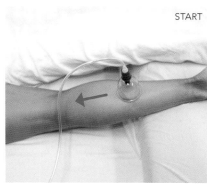

START

▸ The starting point is above the Achilles tendon, wherever a larger cup can comfortably fit on the calf muscle area, usually in the thickest part of the lower leg.
▸ Attach the cup lightly, then gently lift it away from the body until you feel a slight tension engage.
▸ Move the cup up toward the back of the knee, but end below the soft tissue behind the knee joint (endpoint). Detach the cup here, then return to the starting point. Be sure you end the treatment before the back of the knee (the popliteal fossa) without applying cups here. (See Chapter 5: "Safe Cupping" for more information.)
▸ Repeat this line of movement for a minimum of 3 times but no more than a maximum of 5 times.

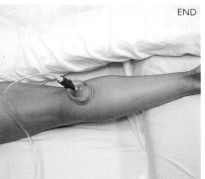

END

When the entire left leg has been addressed, repeat the sequence of Steps 5, 6 and 7 on the right leg.

Next, instruct the person to turn over for work in the supine position.

The Supine Position

The abdomen is the most central part of the body — our core. There is a concentration of lymphatic activity in this region and work here is a vital part of a full body lymphatic drainage treatment. Just the same, working the abdomen can be a very powerful application on its own.

Be sure to treat the abdomen after completing the cupping work to the back of the body (Steps 1 to 8). All the drained lymph material that was deposited along the sides of the body (Steps 1, 2, 5, 6 and half of 7) will be brought through to their primary drainage endpoints, located within the abdomen (the upper inguinal lymph nodes, which are connected to the cisterna chyli, a major lymph drainage vessel that filters lymph up into the termination thoracic ducts, located in the upper chest region).

Remember: If there is an excess of abdominal congestion (such as with constipation), treat this area first for constipation and then begin the full body sequence.

STEP 9: STARTING THE ABDOMEN

Begin treating the abdomen just above the hip bones (anterior superior iliac spine, or ASIS); this stimulates the upper inguinal lymph nodes to receive lymph from the midsection.

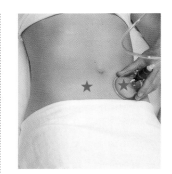

▸ The starting point is just above the ASIS hip points, on the left and right sides of the abdomen respectively.

▸ To locate it, place the fingertips on either hip bone, then mark a diagonal line up toward the navel. The point is between the ASIS hip bone and navel, in the middle of the imaginary line drawn between the two points, located above the hip bones and slightly to the left and right respectively.

▸ Attach the cup, then gently use the lift-and-release technique for a minimum of 3 times but no more than a maximum of 5 times in the same location.

▸ This stimulates the upper inguinal lymph node area.

Repeat this sequence on the right side of the body.

STEP 10: THE ABDOMEN

Begin addressing the abdomen in the lower region, just above the anterior superior iliac spine, or ASIS.

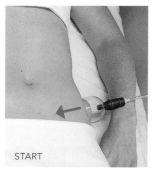

START

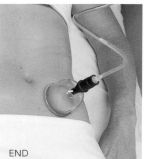

END

▸ The starting point is along the side of the body (shown right), the endpoints for Step 1 from the back of the body; this is located just above the hip bones along the side of the body, where you may rest your hands when standing.

▸ Attach the cup lightly, then gently lift it away from the body until you feel a slight tension engage.

▸ Move the cup from the outside of the body in toward the lower abdomen; this endpoint is exactly where the cup was applied in Step 9. Detach cup here, then return to the starting point.

▸ Repeat each line of movement for a minimum of 3 times but no more than a maximum of 5 times.

▸ Progress your way up the abdomen, one cup width at a time; place the second cup directly above the first cup's line of movement and progress up the rib cage until you are below the breast tissue.

▸ End treating the abdomen just below the breast tissue.

Breast tissue: Licensed professionals with proper lymph drainage training may choose to also drain breast tissue at this point in the treatment. This is done at the discretion of the person working with the cups, as well as the comfort of the person receiving the work. If choosing to treat this area, drainage is out toward the axilla (armpit).

Repeat this sequence on the right side of the abdomen.

When both sides of the abdomen are finished, use the cup to gently follow the entire colon's anatomy 2 or 3 times. This is done with light and lymphatic intentions, so the sectional details need not be as precise as the application for constipation outlined in Chapter 8. Rather, move the cup in a clockwise circle very lightly around the abdomen, starting with the ascending colon (lower right side of abdomen) and ending below the navel (over the rectum region).

Refer to the application for constipation in Chapter 8, page 178, for anatomical direction of the colon if need be. The colon starts in the lower right abdomen, travels up toward the right side of the rib cage (ascending colon), across the abdomen toward the left side of the rib cage (transverse colon), down toward the left hip bones (descending colon) and then bends back toward the midline, finishing about one hand's width below the belly button (sigmoid colon and rectum).

Next, treat the front of the thigh (shown bottom right).

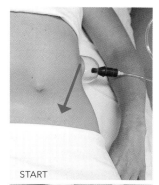

START

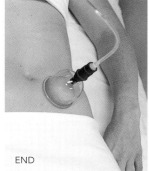

END

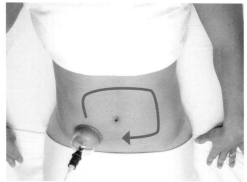

STEP 11: THE UPPER THIGH

Begin addressing the front of the leg by addressing the upper inner thigh; this stimulates the lower inguinal lymph nodes to receive lymph from the leg.

▸ The starting point is about one hand's width from the groin, along the medial half of the upper thigh.
▸ Attach the cup, then gently use the lift-and-release technique for a minimum of 3 times but no more than a maximum of 5 times in this area.

Note

The cup does not need to be all the way up into the groin area — the femoral triangle. (See Chapter 5: "Safe Cupping" for more information.) Lymph can be processed from a comfortable distance, about a hand width's distance from the groin area.

STEP 12: THE FRONT OF THE THIGH

Begin treating the front of the thigh just above the knee.

▸ The starting point is above the knee, starting along the inside of the thigh.

▸ Attach the cup lightly, then gently lift it away from the body until you feel a slight tension engage.

▸ Move the cup up at a slight angle toward the upper inner thigh — where the cup was applied in Step 11. Detach the cup here, then return to the starting point.

Note

This may be a very sensitive line of movement, so use the lift-and-release technique to move over this area comfortably if necessary.

▸ Repeat this line of movement for a minimum of 3 times but no more than a maximum of 5 times.

▸ Address the entire thigh like this, progressing one cup width at a time across the top of the thigh and ending along the outer thigh. Each line of movement will start above the knee and end at the same endpoints (Step 11 points).

Next, treat the front lower leg.

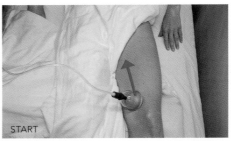
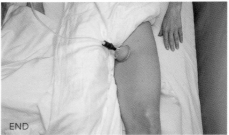
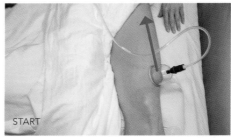
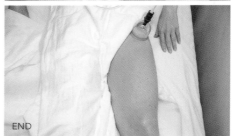

STEP 13: (OPTIONAL) FRONT OF THE LOWER LEG

Smaller cups are needed to work this area.

Begin addressing the front of the lower leg just above the ankle. Address the inside of the leg first, then the outside. Split the front of the lower leg in half lengthwise, around the tibia (shin bone). The inner line will go along the inside of the shin bone toward the knee; the outer line will go along the outside of the shin bone toward the knee.

▸ The starting point is above the ankle, wherever a larger cup will comfortably fit on the front lower leg area.

Note

This may be a very sensitive line of movement, so use the lift-and-release technique to move over this area comfortably if necessary.

▸ Attach the cup lightly, then gently lift it away from the body until you feel a slight tension engage.
▸ Move the cup up toward the knee, ending below the inside of the knee (endpoint). Detach the cup here, then return to the starting point.
▸ Repeat this line of movement for a minimum of 3 times but no more than a maximum of 5 times.

Repeat this sequence on the outer line.

Repeat the sequence of Steps 11, 12 and 13 on the right leg.

Next, treat the upper extremity.

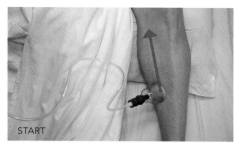
START

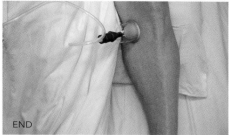
END

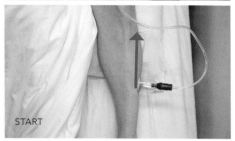
START

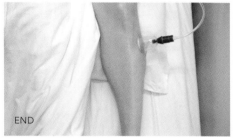
END

STEP 14: THE OUTER CHEST AND AXILLA REGION

Begin addressing the arm by targeting the outer chest region, just outside the armpit; this stimulates the lymph nodes located around the axilla region to receive lymph from the arm. If there is excessive congestion, you may *very lightly* — barely any suction at all — apply the lift-and-release technique 3 to 5 times directly in the armpit.

▸ The starting point is at the edge of the chest, before the armpit begins.
▸ To locate it, place fingertips just in the crease where the armpit begins on the front of the shoulder. Place the cup just medial (inside) to this edge, on the chest tissue. Be sure this placement is above breast tissue.
▸ Attach the cup, then gently use the lift-and-release technique for a minimum of 3 times but no more than a maximum of 5 times in the same location.

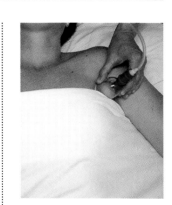

STEP 15: THE UPPER ARM

Begin addressing the upper arm just above the elbow.

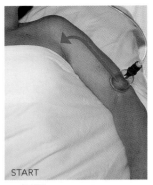

START

▸ The starting point is above the elbow joint, wherever a larger cup will comfortably fit on the upper arm.

▸ Attach the cup lightly, then gently lift it away from the body until you feel a slight tension engage.

Note

This may be a sensitive line of movement or difficult to traverse because of tight muscles, so use the lift-and-release technique to move over this area comfortably if necessary.

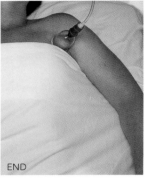

▸ Move the cup in toward the body, then turn slightly once the arm meets the body and finish just outside the axilla (armpit), where the cup was applied in Step 14.

▸ Detach the cup here, then return to the starting point.

▸ Repeat this line of movement for a minimum of 3 times but no more than a maximum of 5 times in the same exact location.

Next, treat the lower arm, same side.

END

Drainage of Lower Arm Is Optional

This application is not required when doing a full body treatment. It may be useful to drain the lower arm if you are addressing the arm (for example, for carpal tunnel syndrome). Addressing the upper arm will directly benefit the drainage of the lower arm — clearing a proximal area before a distal one has a direct effect on distal lymphatic drainage activity.

STEP 16: THE LOWER ARM

Smaller cups are required to work this area.

Begin addressing the lower arm just above the wrist. Split the lower arm in half — the outside (posterior) and inside (anterior). Treat the outside of the forearm first, then the inside.

▸ The starting point is above the wrist, wherever a larger cup will comfortably fit on the front of the lower arm.

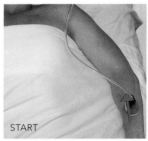

START

Note

This may be a very sensitive line of movement and a vascular area, so use light suction and the recommended lift-and-release technique to move over this area comfortably if necessary.

▸ Attach the cup lightly, then gently lift it away from the body until you feel a slight tension engage.

▸ Move the cup up toward the elbow, ending below the elbow joint (endpoint). Detach the cup here, then return to the starting point.

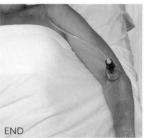

END

- Repeat this line of movement for a minimum of 3 times but no more than a maximum of 5 times.
- Repeat this sequence from the outside to the inside (anterior) side of the forearm.

Repeat the sequence of Steps 14, 15 and 16 on the right arm.

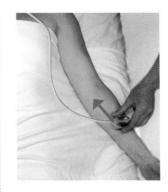

Safety Point

There are many superficial blood vessels in this area, so work mindfully. (See Chapter 5: "Safe Cupping" for more information about working with vascular considerations.)

The Upper Chest: Endpoint of Full Body Cupping Sequence

There is a concentration of lymphatic activity in this region, which surrounds the major thoracic drainage ducts. It is very important to address this section after completing the work to the rest of the body.

STEP 17: THE UPPER CHEST

Begin addressing the upper chest just below the clavicle (collarbones).

- The starting point is in the midline of the chest, below the clavicle but above the breast tissue.
- Attach the cup, then gently lift it away from the chest until you feel a slight tension engage.
- Slowly move the cup out toward the axilla (armpit), ending just before the crease into the underarm (endpoint). Detach the cup here, then return to the starting point.

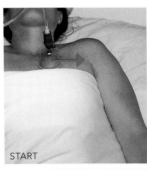

START

Note

This may be a sensitive line of movement; use the lift-and-release technique to treat this area if necessary.

- Repeat this line of movement a minimum of 3 times but no more than a maximum of 5 times.
- End addressing the upper chest out by the axilla (armpit).

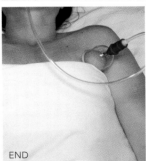

END

Repeat this sequence on the right side of the upper chest.

This completes the full body lymphatic drainage treatment.

FACE AND HEAD LYMPHATIC DRAINAGE

Note

It is highly recommended you use a set of cups specific for this type of work. These cups are designed for the small features of the face as well as the delicate, easy-to-mark, face tissue.

The head is an area of the body that encounters a lot of congestion. Whether it is sinus congestion, facial tension or overall head congestion (in the case of head injuries), gentle cupping to mimic lymphatic drainage can be very effective and offer relief.

THERAPEUTIC THOUGHT: FACE CUPPING FEEDBACK

One of my clients, who had no particular affliction but wanted to experience the effects of cup work on her face, offered this feedback after treatment: "It feels like you drained the stress out of my face!" Who doesn't want that!?

One of my students, who works in a hospital and applied the therapy to a patient who had suffered a severe head trauma, reported that it was the only therapy that seemed to offer some relief from congestion. The patient was overjoyed and the medical staff, while unfamiliar with the technique, were equally excited about the treatment's effectiveness.

GUIDELINES FOR FACE AND HEAD DRAINAGE

The same basic guidelines that apply to the full body lymphatic drainage (see pages 199 for full detailed descriptions) apply for face and head drainage:

CUPPING 101

Do not push cups into the face. While it may be difficult at times for a cup to adhere or move, avoid pushing it into the tissue. This can be painful and counterproductive.

1. **Pressure should be light.** Attempts to move lymph fluid should be gentle, which is more effective when addressing the drainage pathways of the head than applying strong pressure.
2. **Use moving cups or lift-and-release techniques — no stationary cups.** Use either of these techniques to address the tissue accordingly, or combine the two as you see necessary (a combination technique known as the Morse Code of Cups; see page 110).
3. **Cup should be proportional to the face, sometimes larger in size.** You will want to use appropriate-sized cups depending on the area being treated (cheek versus upper lip).
4. **Movements should be slow, rhythmic, repetitive.** The intent is to treat surface tissue rather than anything deeper.
5. **Treat the entire face evenly, one cup width at a time.** Each section should be treated completely, one cup width at a time. For example, a larger forehead may need three or four cup widths; others may only accommodate two. Furthermore, every step's line of movement will be repeated for a minimum of 3 times but no more than a maximum of 5 times, ensuring a universal, even treatment.

6. **Treat and drain more proximal regions before attempting distal areas.** Just as with the full body, the face needs to be treated in the appropriate, logical manner. Face and head drainage should begin at the neck, then progress up the length of the face.
7. **Note the direction for drainage.** See page 201 for step-by-step instruction, along with detailed directions for the flow of drainage. Be sure to follow it to the best of your ability.
8. **Use only the lift-and-release technique in the front of the neck — no moving cups.** Remember that this is an endangerment site and vascular damage can occur. (See Chapter 5: "Safe Cupping" for more information.)
9. **Work one side of the face at a time.** Begin with the left side of the neck and face. Divide the face in half, left to right. Once a section has been cupped, on the left side address the right side unless otherwise specified (for example, between Steps 5 and 6, and Steps 9, 10 & 11, page 223, where you do not change sides).

Note

Unfortunately, facial hair will not allow the small cups to adhere to the skin, even with a good amount of oil applied to the skin. The thinner the facial hair — for example, one day without shaving — the easier it may be to attach a cup.

Before You Begin

Clean the skin and have a good-quality face oil ready to use. It can be a premium esthetic-grade face massage oil or a naturally light food-grade oil, such as coconut, avocado, extra-virgin olive oil or any other low-fragrance oil, that can smoothly slide over the skin. Apply an ample amount of oil to the skin (not dripping), wipe off hands and pick up the face cup attached to the squeeze bulb.

Body Position

Face and head lymphatic drainage works best with some elevation of the head. For self-care, position a mirror so you are able to watch what you are doing. Stay standing or seated, whatever is most comfortable. When applying cups to someone else, the person can be lying down on their back, perhaps with a small pillow under their head for slight elevation if excess congestion is present, although the elevation is not necessary.

Techniques to Use

- Use only the lift-and-release technique in the anterior neck or the Universal Pass (see page 219).
- Moving cups can be used for most of the face. If these are uncomfortable or difficult to slide, the lift-and-release technique may be used anywhere on the face. Use a combined style of sliding and lift-and-release techniques if necessary.
- Use only the lift-and-release technique in Steps 9 and 10, the areas directly next to the eye.

For detailed, step-by-step instructions on how to use each suggested technique, see pages 107 to 111 in Chapter 7: "Using Cups in Treatment."

STEP 1: INITIAL PLACEMENTS

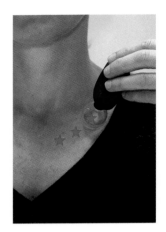

▸ Begin by applying a larger face cup just under the clavicle (collar bone). Using the lift-and-release technique, apply it to three points (shown left) just off the side in the center of the chest, progressing out toward the armpit. This series of lift-and-release cupping prepares the region to drain from the face and down the neck (unclog the drain).

▸ The starting point is just below (about 1 finger's width) the clavicle in the midline of the body where it attaches to the sternum.

▸ To locate it, place the *opposite hand's* index finger on the clavicle in the center of the chest, where it connects to the sternum; if palpating the left clavicle, use your right index finger. Slide your finger just below the clavicle (about 1 finger's width below, there will be a slight soft tissue divot about the length of your finger along the bottom edge of the collarbone). This soft tissue space is the line of application, and the starting point is at the centermost space where the clavicle meets the sternum and the soft tissue space begins. Be sure the line of application is *below* the clavicle, not touching the bone with the cup.

▸ Apply a cup to the first point in the middle just below the clavicle, using the lift-and-release once, move the cup one cup's width over toward the shoulder and apply the lift-and-release technique again, then move the cup over one more cup's width and apply the lift-and-release again, completing three location points in all.

▸ The location of the third cup's placement will be the endpoint for every completed section and for every Universal Pass (discussed later, after Step 1) thereafter.

Repeat this sequence on the right side of the face.

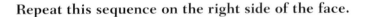

Beginning of Lymph Drainage Sequence

To start the drainage process, begin by addressing the front of the neck in the anterior triangle region. There is a high concentration of lymph nodes in this region (some of these are the lymph nodes that get swollen when you are sick and are easy to palpate), therefore, clearing this region helps prepare for the reception of any drained lymph moving down from the face and neck.

STEP 2: THE ANTERIOR TRIANGLE/FRONT OF THE NECK

ONLY THE LIFT-AND-RELEASE TECHNIQUE is used in this entire section — the anterior triangle (See Chapter 5: "Safe Cupping" for more information.)

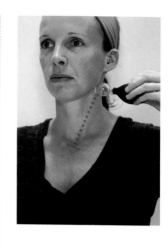

- The starting point is below the ear and the jawline, in the soft tissue space of the front of the neck.
- Use the lift-and-release application down the front side of the neck, following a slight diagonal line toward the midline of the chest and ending just below the clavicle — this is the same endpoint as in Step 1: Initial Placements and for the rest of the face treatment. This line goes over the sternocleidomastoid (SCM) muscle of the front neck.
- A longer neck may need four lift-and-release placements; a shorter neck may require three.
- 1st pass, go directly over the SCM.
- 2nd pass, go slightly (one cup's width) behind it.
- 3rd pass, go slightly (one cup's width) behind the 2nd pass.
- Repeat this line of movement (down the front side of the neck, around the clavicle and finishing at the endpoint under the clavicle — the same endpoint as in Step 1: Initial Placement) multiple times; a minimum of 6 passes but not more than a maximum of 9 passes. For individuals with more congestion or those who are receiving this application for the first time, it is recommended to do 9 passes to adequately clear and stimulate the lymphatic drainage process. Picture this line of movement as an L, for moving lymph.

REPEATING THE UNIVERSAL PASS

- This is a repeated and required drainage pass that travels diagonally down the side of the neck.
- The Universal Pass needs to be done only once after every step is completed; this ensures a continuous drain down the neck and into the chest.
- The Universal Pass is simply one draining pass of lift-and-release down the side of the neck — exactly the same as the first line of movement in Step 2.

STEP 3: JUST UNDER THE CHIN

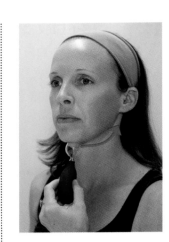

Apply one larger face cup just under the jawline, starting at the center of the face under the chin. In general, one cup width and line of movement will suffice; however, if someone has more under-chin tissue (for example, a double chin), you may use 2 or 3 lines of movement to complete this section.

▸ The starting point is under the chin. Attach the cup lightly here; the cup will be angled up toward the face. You will be working underneath the chin and progressing along the underside of the jawline. Once the cup is attached, gently lift it away from the skin until you feel a slight tension engage, then slide the cup along the skin, using either a moving cup or lift-and-release technique to complete this line of movement.
▸ The line of movement is from the midline of the chin, along the underside of the jaw, ending under the jawline and straight below the ear (this endpoint is where you will start the Universal Pass). Detach the cup here, then return to the starting point.

Note

A moving cup in this section should not be considered within the anterior triangle but rather along the underside of the chin and jawbone.

When section is completed, repeat the Universal Pass once. Repeat the Universal Pass once.

Repeat this sequence on the right side of the face.

STEP 4: ALONG THE JAWLINE, UNDER THE LIP

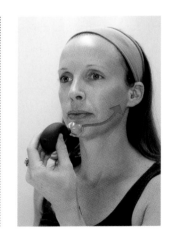

▸ The starting point is in the midline on the chin and just below the lower lip.
▸ The line of movement is along the chin and jawline toward the ear, over the lower cheek and ending just in front of the earlobe (endpoint). Detach the cup here, then return to the starting point.

When section is completed, repeat the Universal Pass once.

Repeat this sequence on the right side of the face.

STEP 5: UPPER LIP

A very small cup is used here. Do not include the actual lip tissue.

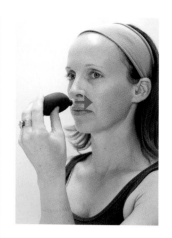

▸ The starting point is in the midline of the upper lip, under the nose but above the lip tissue.

▸ The line of movement is very small, from the center of the tissue above the lip but below the nose, then over to the side of the mouth where the lip ends (endpoint).

▸ Every upper lip is different, so sliding may be difficult due to anatomical contours or any slight facial hair (this will not work over mustaches or beards). Detach the cup here, then return to the starting point.

There is no need for the Universal Pass after Step 5. Proceed to Step 6, same side of face, then the Universal Pass.

STEP 6: CHEEK REGION

Begin this step immediately after completing Step 5, the same side of the face (shown right), where Step 5 ended, at the edge of the upper lip and in the cheek tissue. This area may accommodate two or three cup widths, depending on the length of the cheek.

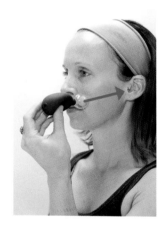

▸ The starting point is at the edge of the upper lip, one cup's width above the corner of mouth, where Step 5 ended.

▸ The line of movement is along the cheek toward the ear, ending just in front of the ear (endpoint). Detach the cup here, then return to the starting point.

▸ The cup may pop off when you pass over the temporomandibular joint (TMJ) area of the jaw due to tight muscles; address this tightness, perhaps with the TMJD basic application (see page 187), and continue to the endpoint.

▸ Cupping the area at the starting point alongside the nose (2nd line of movement shown here) is an effective bonus treatment for sinus congestion (see the basic application for sinus congestion on page 190 for more details on this exact location). If desired, apply the lift-and-release technique 2 or 3 times — or apply a stationary cup for a maximum of 10 seconds here — then follow the line of movement along the cheek towards the ear.

When section is completed, repeat the Universal Pass once.

Repeat the sequence of Steps 5 and 6 to the right side of the face.

Notes
Step 5 ends when the upper rim of the cup is just below the delicate eye tissue region.

STEP 7: THE CENTER LINE OF THE FOREHEAD

This area of the face contributes to sinus drainage. While Step 6 began the sinus-opening process, this step continues it. The movement here is up toward the hairline. This both soothes forehead tension and encourages drainage up toward the sagittal suture at the top of the head (the centerline where to cranial bones meet, top of the skull) and away from the area of high congestion between the eyebrows.

▸ The starting point is the space between the eyebrows.
▸ The line of movement is straight up the forehead toward the hairline (endpoint). Detach the cup here, then return to the starting point.

Note

Foreheads may contain a lot of tension and therefore a moving cup may be a challenge. If so, use the lift-and-release technique to complete lines of movement in Steps 7 and 8.

There is no need to repeat the Universal Pass after this step. Continue to Step 8, same side of face.

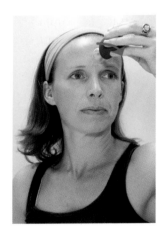

STEP 8: THE FOREHEAD

▸ The starting point is in the midline of the forehead at the hairline where Step 7 ended.
▸ The line of movement is from the midline of the forehead out toward the sides of the forehead, stopping just in front of the hairline in the temporal region. Detach the cup here, then return to the center line starting points.
▸ You will be progressing your way *down the forehead* toward the eyebrow. This section may accommodate two or three cup widths, depending on the length of the forehead; a larger forehead could accommodate three or four cup widths.

Safety Point

Skip over any obvious blood vessels here, such as a protruding temporal artery. Sliding a cup across blood vessels can cause damage.

When section is completed, repeat the Universal Pass once.

Repeat this sequence on the right side of the face.

STEP 9: UNDER THE EYE REGION

Very small cups with very light suction are used.

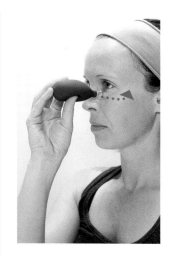

▸ The starting point is near the nose and under the eyelashes, outside of the eye itself.
▸ Apply the cup very gently.
▸ *Use only the lift-and-release technique.* Do not add the extra tension lift to the tissue when the cup is applied, so as to not stretch this extra-delicate skin.
▸ Progress the gentle cupping work out toward the temporal region, using about 3 or 4 cup placements.

There is no need to repeat the Universal Pass after this section. Continue to Step 10, the upper eye on the same side of the face.

STEP 10: ABOVE THE EYE REGION

Very small cups with very light suction are used.

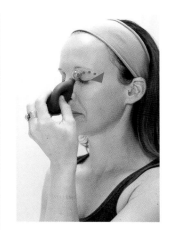

▸ The starting point is near the nose and under the eyebrow, above the eyelid.
▸ Attach the cup, then apply a very gentle lift-and-release technique and move it out toward the temporal region, using about 3 or 4 cup placements. Do not add the extra tension lift to the tissue when the cup is applied so it will not stretch this extra-delicate skin.

There is no need to repeat the Universal Pass after this section. Continue to Step 11, the eyebrow region on the same side of the face.

STEP 11: THE EYEBROW

▸ The starting point is directly over the eyebrow, at the midline of the face where the eyebrow begins.
▸ The line of movement is along the entire eyebrow, starting from the midline and progressing out toward the outer edge of the eyebrow.

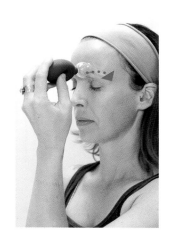

Note

Thicker eyebrows or bony orbital ridge contours may pose a challenge for this step. If so, repeat this application on the bottommost line of Step 7 (the forehead).

When section is completed, repeat the Universal Pass once.

Repeat Steps 9, 10 and 11 on the right side of face.

This completes the entire face and head drainage treatment.

Chapter 10
Advanced Applications

ADVANCED APPLICATIONS OF THERAPEUTIC CUPPING

By now you know that therapeutic cupping is an incredibly diverse form of bodywork. From common applications for soft tissue and muscle discomforts (Chapter 8) to light and lymphatic applications (Chapter 9), the practice of cupping can be as varied as the person using it. Some applications of cups are more advanced than others, however, and require more attention to detail. In this chapter, some of these more complex conditions and/or applications will be discussed and demonstrated. Inflammation, for example, is a complicated condition that can benefit from cupping, but there are various stages of inflammation, as well as contributing factors — such as injuries or autoimmune system dysfunction — that require proper knowledge and assessment in order to safely and effectively apply treatment with cups. Cupping during pregnancy is also possible, but it needs to be approached with much care and a thorough understanding of the body at every phase of pregnancy before it is attempted. Scar tissue, sports recovery, pulmonary conditions and cellulite all respond positively to cupping. Yet again, each application used to treat them varies greatly from the next and understanding the anatomy, potential restrictions and safety concerns relevant to each case is crucial for optimal results.

WORKING WITH INFLAMMATION: ACUTE VERSUS CHRONIC

Inflammation generally occurs in any area where there is an injury or infection. Initial inflammatory responses work to stabilize the site, remove any waste materials (such as damaged tissue) via lymphatic drainage and initiate the healing process. This is a necessary component of any tissue repair and a crucial part of healthy bodily functions. Therapeutic cupping can be used to help reduce inflammation as well as assist in the overall healing process inflammation initiates.

Inflammation can be categorized as acute or chronic, depending on its duration and underlying cause. Chronic inflammation of the shoulder joint, for example, can be due to an old injury that never fully healed, and chronic inflammation of the knee joint can occur because of an autoimmune condition such as rheumatoid arthritis. Modified applications of cupping can help with the removal of waste materials from the location of acute inflammation and help relieve chronic inflammation when applied directly over the site. When addressing soft tissue inflammation, make sure that the line between acute and chronic is clear and always work within the recipient's comfort zone, as this area can be sensitive.

In this section, the focus will be on inflammation due to musculoskeletal injuries — joint or soft tissue damages — rather than inflammation associated with viral or bacterial infections. Inflammation of musculoskeletal injuries are easier to approach with cups, whereas viral or bacterial-related inflammations require more specific medical diagnosis and attention.

It is important to be able to recognize when an area is injured and inflamed. The *four primary characteristics of trauma-related inflammation* are swelling, redness, pain and decreased function.

- When trauma occurs, the body releases histamines, which cause blood vessels to dilate and allows healing tissue fluids to flood the injured area, resulting in swelling.
- With increased local circulation, extra plasma is drawn into the area and increase *heat and redness*.
- As the pressure increases, the nerve endings (nociceptors) in the dermis start to fire, resulting in *pain*.
- The sum of all these contributing factors ultimately limits range of motion and *decreases function* of the area.

Chemical processes that occur during an acute inflammatory response include:

- The release of cytokines ("emergency alert" cells) begins the response process.
- This stimulates the release of white blood cells, platelets, fibroblasts (the "rebuilders") and other healing chemicals into the bloodstream, or plasma.
- As this enriched plasma fills the traumatized area, the white blood cells begin the processes of phagocytosis (cell eating) and pinocytosis (cell drinking) in which they engulf and remove damaged cellular debris, foreign objects and any other unwelcome pathogenic material.
- The plasma cleanses the area with a flushing-like action, thereby diluting any acidic or toxic substances in the trauma site.
- The waste material is then transported to lymphatic system to be removed.
- Clotting proteins begin to seal any breaks in the damaged structures, and the process of regeneration begins thereafter.

Categories of Inflammation

Understanding the difference between acute and chronic inflammation is imperative before using cups. The type of inflammation and relative state of the person's health will influence your work with cups, so be sure to understand the full scope of any condition — a proper diagnosis, assessment of the condition and knowing how long the inflammation has been present in the area are all important. If someone has one of the more complicated conditions — for example, a severe sprain or chronic systemic inflammation — exercise caution when applying cups (or refer to a specialized bodyworker) so you are less likely to cause (more) damage.

Acute inflammation is an immediate response to injury or infection. The body's reaction can be almost instant and usually lasts a few days, though in some instances it may last longer. Acute inflammation can also describe the period when chronic inflammatory conditions (lupus, some cases of fibromyalgia, asthma, Crohn's disease, rheumatoid arthritis, etc.) flare up and exacerbate any dormant symptoms, such as intensifying any relative pain, dysfunction or swelling.

Chronic inflammation is more complicated and can last anywhere from a few weeks to years, depending on what is causing the response. Chronic inflammation can reside in a joint (such as chronic knee pain) or be associated with an autoimmune disorder. This dysfunction can be caused by either the body's inability to dispose of whatever caused the acute inflammation, constant low-grade inflammation that never fully dissipates or an autoimmune response, when the body attacks healthy tissue because it mistakenly identifies perfectly healthy tissue as pathogenic, bringing about a constant inflammatory response.

Joint Inflammation

Inflammation most commonly occurs within the more mobile joints of the body: slightly mobile (amphiarthrotic) joints, such as vertebrae and freely moving (diarthrotic) joints, like the knee. The term "arthritis" is often used to describe most joint inflammations and can occur within any joint structure: the synovial membranes, the joint capsule, bursae, ligaments or even the periosteum of the bone. Whether from direct trauma, repetitive motion — wear and tear — injuries (osteoarthritis) or autoimmune dysfunction (rheumatoid arthritis), arthritic joints respond well to therapeutic cupping.

Soft Tissue Inflammation

Of the human body's many tissues (from bone to epithelial tissue), muscles and tendons are considered one of the strongest, yet they are vulnerable structures that go through a lot of repetitive exertions and stress — a perfect setting for potential injury and inflammation. Inflammation within these structures can vary tremendously. Low-grade inflammation can occur from repetitive wear and tear like regular exercise routines, while high-grade inflammation can be caused by a traumatic injury like severe strains to muscles or tendons.

While the most common care for strains is rest, ice, compression and elevation, this protocol can (literally) freeze the lymphatic system, thus hindering the recovery process. Allowing the body to do its work at the site of injury and then supporting the removal of waste within the lymphatic system with the use of cupping can assist the healing process. This is an action that requires the movement of bodily fluids, and it should be allowed to keep moving, rather than being 'frozen' in place.

Systemic Inflammation

System inflammatory conditions, such as lupus or fibromyalgia, are very complicated, yet they share the common denominator of inflammation. For conditions like lupus, which affects most joints and surrounding tissue, or fibromyalgia, often generalized as overall, undefined systemic inflammation, therapeutic cupping can offer impressive relief when applied in a more superficial, overall application. Consider using cups to dissipate such inflammation, utilizing a full body lymphatic drainage in such cases. See Chapter 9: "Therapeutic Cupping for Lymphatic Drainage," for more information.

ACUTE INFLAMMATION AND CUPPING

The purpose of acute inflammation is to stabilize injured tissue and begin the healing process. The lymphatic system will naturally help remove inflammatory waste materials from the injured area, but this process may be challenged at this stage because the injured tissue may impair drainage. This is where cups can help. By properly directing the drainage, cups help facilitate the "flushing" process inherently performed by the lymphatic system. Tight tissues inhibit natural lymph drainage, but with applied *negative* pressure, cups can create a more open channel for fluids to move within the layers of tissue. Also, lymph fluids have little to no natural directional guidance within the superficial lymphatic system, so cups can easily influence the path of drainage — wherever the cup moves, fluid follows it. Considering all of these factors, gentle control of suction pressure and direction of drainage is imperative.

> **DID YOU KNOW?**
>
> Tendonitis, or tendinitis (inflammation injury of a tendon), and tendinosis (degenerative injury of a tendon without inflammation) are different conditions and should be diagnosed accordingly. Tendonitis is a more acute case of inflammation, while tendinosis is considered chronic.

Safety Point

Wait *at least* 72 hours after the first signs of inflammation occur before attempting to gently begin this supported clearing process. The more severe the injury, the longer the acute phase may last.

Note

When addressing acute or chronic inflammation, it is important to work in the direction lymph naturally drains. Refer to Chapter 9: "Therapeutic Cupping for Lymphatic Drainage" for more information.

Where to Place Cups

Perhaps the most important thing to remember here is to work *proximal* to the area of inflammation only — that is, next/closer to the attachment point — not *directly* on the inflamed area. Placing cups directly over inflamed tissue would, by nature, draw more fluid into the area and create excessive swelling, potentially damaging the very tissue the body is trying to stabilize and repair.

Let's take the example of a recent knee replacement, 6 weeks after surgery, with swelling in the general area of the knee. Here's how to approach a cupping treatment:

▶ Use light suction pressure and apply either the lift-and-release or moving cups (not stationary) technique *above* the knee, in the thigh region.

▶ Attach the cup *above the knee (proximal)*, about a hand's width away from the knee joint.

▶ Lift the cup very gently away from the thigh until you feel a slight tension engage.

▶ Slowly and gently move the cup toward the groin, always maintaining a comfortable suction.

▶ Repeat these lines of movement — front of the thigh up toward the groin *and* back of the thigh (if possible, depending on the person's position and comfort level) up toward the hips — for a maximum of 5 times but no less than a minimum of 3 times. Remember, if a moving cup is too sensitive, switch to a lift-and-release technique, or mix the two as needed (known as the Morse Code of Cups; see page 110).

▶ It is recommended to apply a few lift-and-release applications near the lower inguinal lymph nodes (just below the groin area) to help stimulate the overall process of regional drainage.

This basic application can quickly, safely and effectively drain inflammation from the knee. The body will then continue its cycle of cleaning and repairing with less interstitial waste fluid obstructing the progress.

CHRONIC INFLAMMATION AND CUPPING

Understanding the chronic inflammatory condition is important before cupping the area. Colitis (chronic inflammation of the colon), for example, is approached completely differently from arthritis in the elbow, just as bursitis in the hip is treated differently from chronic knee inflammation. The only common denominator when treating all chronic inflammatory conditions with cups is that you *can* place cups *directly* over the site of the inflammation.

Chronic inflammation needs to be addressed initially by flushing out the area in a similar manner as with flushing out acute inflammation (following the drainage pathway directions), but with chronic inflammation, cups placed directly over these areas can yield significant relief. In an optimally functioning body, soft tissue is hydrated, pliable and circulating regular tissue fluids. A body with chronic inflammation, however, contains heat that can literally dry out layers of soft tissue. Any trapped or embedded inflammation can contribute to restrictions of these tissues, from dehydrated muscles to fused fascial adhesions to restricted joint mobility. If chronic inflammation and its heat are not removed, there can be a perpetual state of unhealthy tissue. Therefore, the simultaneous responses of enhanced vasodilation, the vacuum drawing out of inflammatory materials, and the decompression of potentially fused, dehydrated tissue are welcome therapeutic benefits unique to cupping.

Let's take the example of chronic knee pain, with 5 years of pain and recurring inflammation. Here's how to approach a cupping treatment:

- Begin by following the same suggested application as with acute inflammation, initiating the clearing process.
- For the knee joint, use smaller cups (see the Primary Application for knee problems in Chapter 8, page 171, for suggestions on how to approach this area).
- Stationary cups (or the lift-and-release technique if stationary cups are too sensitive on initial applications) can be placed around the knee joint, and suction pressure can vary according to the person's comfort — light, medium or strong.
- Allow the cups to remain for a maximum of 3 minutes and a minimum of 30 seconds. You may see a variety of colors and temperatures come to the surface (whether marking tissue or offering a type of "looking glass" into the anatomy with temporary marks that may show underlying stagnations) in such a small, condensed area.
- After working directly on the knee, repeat the same clearing process that you started with.

ATHLETIC PERFORMANCE AND CUPPING

Cups have been used for years in sports training and rehabilitation. The intense physical exertions during training and competitive events require a higher level of performance from muscles, which in turn can produce an increase in the volume of heat and metabolic waste, such as lactic acid. Some of the most important benefits from cupping involve muscle recovery, manipulation and forced hydration into these overexerted muscles.

Athletes are used to having their bodies manipulated and receiving all sorts of bodywork to keep them performing at their best, so cupping can be easily introduced into their training regimen. Using cups on a regular basis can help maintain healthier muscles, which in turn can aid in preventing injury. Many trainers already employ cupping, a technique they often refer to as myofascial decompression, or MFD.

Muscle Activity in Athletes

What happens inside the muscle tissue of an athlete is more intense than that of the average person, mainly the process of energy production. Whether using aerobic or anaerobic metabolism (See "Muscular System," page 50 for more information on aerobic and anaerobic metabolism) to access energy, athletes make higher demands of their muscles and, in doing so, create more waste. Waste products like heat and lactic acid, as well as other cellular by-products like protons — the "garbage" from the broken-down adenosine triphosphate (ATP) — all occur in great quantities within an athlete's muscles. Muscles naturally try to expel these wastes via lymph drainage, but disposal is often challenged because of the athlete's tight and toned muscles.

Anatomy FYI

Adenosine triphosphate (ATP) is an energy-producing substance in the body that is used to carry out countless cellular activities, including the production of energy necessary for muscle contractions. During muscle energy production, the body uses either oxygen or glucose (through aerobic or anaerobic metabolism) to access and release ATP. After its energy is used, ATP's cellular waste substances, such as protons, carbon dioxide, methane and acetate, are systematically recycled, ultimately replenishing the body's supply of ATP.

Athletes' Muscle Recovery

Considering that these strongly developed muscles must be continually ready to train and perform, a quick recovery time is very important. Muscles need to usher out waste products quickly and allow healthy blood and oxygen to return, over and over again. Various methods of physical therapy and bodywork can facilitate this process.

Muscle Recovery and Cupping

Cupping can amplify the process of general waste removal required for faster muscle recovery. Cups stimulate the internal flushing mechanism within muscle tissue — a sort of suction pump — thereby accelerating the return of lactate into circulation and welcoming more oxygen into the muscle, which promotes an overall healthier muscle tissue environment. The enhanced exchange of fluids allows for a higher output of energy without exhausting the muscle, yet allows the body more time to recover naturally. Equally beneficial, the negative pressure vacuum of cups draws out metabolic waste, stagnant blood and heat from within the layers of muscle tissue and brings them up to the lymphatic system on the surface for disposal. Allowing heat to escape protects the tissue from getting too hot, which could otherwise create internal inflammation and related damages.

Repetitive Motion Injuries and Athletes

Repetitive motion injuries can happen to anyone who practices activities with repetitive motions, such as hairstylists or golfers. In sports, repetitive motion injuries are very common and can easily inhibit performance. Cupping not only helps facilitate a speedy recovery, but it also potentially prevents these injuries from happening.

When a group of muscles performs the same movements over and over, such as pitching a baseball, it tends to get incredibly tight and restricted. The heat generated as waste can make muscles — such as the rotator cuff, if we stick to the baseball example — more likely to dehydrate and stick together, forming adhesions. These adhesions can bury themselves deeper and deeper into the body if left untreated. While the body will find a way to continue functioning, its performance may diminish — full muscle usage, range of motion and function will be affected. If left untreated, these now drier muscle tissues will continue this vicious cycle of dehydration and adhesions, and potentially tear.

Cupping to Prevent Repetitive Motion Injuries

Providing a continuously healthy muscle environment can prevent injuries before they start. Cups force hydration into these much-used tissues while simultaneously dispelling the trapped heat — out with the bad, in with the good. This timely exchange enables the muscles to remain softer, more flexible and able to go on with high-performance.

Let's continue with the example of baseball pitchers. They use one arm, countlessly repeating intensely exertive movements that require the same muscles and tendons to throw the ball at intense speeds at a specific target. This high-velocity friction in the muscles causes an excess of heat in the tissue and, if not expelled, can cause inflammation and dry out the tissue at the deepest levels, especially in the small space of the shoulder joint. Over time, this continuous low-grade inflammation can settle deep into muscles, maybe even down to the bone, and contribute to a wide range of dysfunction, such as frozen shoulder or rotator cuff muscle damage.

Hydration

Hydration is a vital component of cupping therapy. Cups pull fluids into layers of tissue that were previously dehydrated, fused or inflamed. This supply of fluids comes from the surrounding cellular spaces and deeper hydrated tissues, leaving the body dehydrated. For this reason, the body needs to be replenished. Drinking plenty of water is essential with cupping treatments.

Pre- and Post-event Therapies

There is a big difference between the type of therapies used before and after a sporting event or competition. Cupping can provide excellent benefits at either time but should be done with grave consideration for what cups are doing to the body. The closer to an event, the less invasive any therapy should be, cups or otherwise.

Pre-event Therapies

When working with an athlete before their sporting event, how cups should be used varies with the treatment's intent and desired results. If the intention is to stretch and warm up the tissue before

Client Work

A colleague who works primarily with professional athletes of all classes (Olympic, American League Baseball, American National Football League) suggests that her clients drink enough water that their urine is clear. The occasional client who may feel crummy after a cupping session usually reports not drinking enough water, but they immediately feel better when they increase to the "clear urine output" level.

Client Work

A colleague shared this story:

I worked on an American Major League Baseball player 6 hours before batting practice pre-game (8 hours before the start of the game) and he claimed to have the best batting practice ever! Using a series of cupping techniques in conjunction with manual therapy, I was able to increase his range of motion and release muscle rigidity prior to the game. The result was freer-moving hips and greater rotation when driving the ball into the outfield. —Stacie Nevelus, licensed massage therapist

exertion, cups can be used to help stretch the tissue from the inside out. Cupping uses the body's own blood flow to hydrate and increase pliability, which allows for easier lift and stretch of the fascia and connective tissue, providing a better stretch of the tissue than manual stretching alone. When vacuum therapy is done before an event, the athlete will notice ease movement and less restriction.

The style of application and duration of treatment should also be considered. Do not use very slow and relaxing applications, nor should you use long cupping durations, since you do not want to stimulate the sympathetic nervous system and relax the body. Pre-event cupping should be limited in time — less time for any stationary cups (consider 1 minute rather than 3 minutes maximum) or less overall session time — and far enough in advance of the event so that muscles can be fully adjusted and ready for action.

Knowing your athlete and how they respond to vacuum therapy work is also vital when working on them before an event. This means you do not introduce this therapy for the first time before any event; incorporate it into their training routine and allow the body time to feel the differences and adjust to it before any pre-event usage.

Post-event Therapies

Using cups on an athlete after a sporting event can enhance the removal of metabolic waste and heat that have built up during physical exertion. At the same time, it is bringing oxygen-rich blood and hydration to further nourish the tissue and aid in the recovery process. Using cups in combination with manual therapy (for example, sports massage or passive stretching applications) on an athlete after their event is an opportunity to eradicate any potential muscle issues that may have occurred. In other words, it can stop the onset of injury before it starts.

Following a sporting event or competition and when the body has cooled down, the following applications can be used:

- A cupping application to address the lymphatic drainage pathways (see Chapter 9 for more information) using long, soothing applications either as a full body treatment or focused on more fatigued areas of the body where there is some discomfort. For example, a marathon runner's lower body may be sorest and require more attention. Because the upper body is also pumping repeatedly during the event, it could also be addressed to a lesser degree.
- Soothing and comfortable stationary cups can offer localized decompression over areas of discomfort or soreness. Be mindful not to use too strong a suction pressure, though, as this could cramp the recently dehydrated muscles or cause spasms when applied too quickly after their repetitive contractions. Allow the body to cool down and rehydrate, and then approach the body with cups. Post-event applications can be for longer periods than pre-event, and moving cups should be used at a slower pace, thereby sedating the nervous system and allowing it to welcome the sensations of recovery.

General Cupping for Athletes

When used regularly, cupping can help prevent injuries. Cumulative work helps maintain healthy muscle tissue from one event to the next, and the more this work is done, the greater the potential for overall muscle health, strength and recovery. Whether it be the same day or within a few days of any event, it is recommended to receive these types of vacuum therapies sooner rather than later — once the athlete has rehydrated and cooled down — so as to keep the cycle of muscle rejuvenation going.

CELLULITE AND CUPPING

The "dimples" that appear with cellulite are not only unsightly but also a sign of stagnation within the body — the result of micro-adhesions that form when the superficial fascia (which connects epidermis to everything inside) gets "sticky," creating pockets where adipose tissue can become stagnant. The body wants to be fluid and pliable, but many contributing factors can cause these micro-adhesions to form: poor diet, lack of optimal hydration and a sedentary lifestyle, such as an office job.

The adipose cells are located within the dermis, which is *just* under the skin's surface. To address the stagnation of adipose cells and sticky fascia, there is no need for deep suction pressure, given their shallow depth. What is required is lighter suction pressure and more vigorous circulation-boosting movements to the area in order to break up the small adhesions without damaging the other structures in this area, such as blood vessels or nerves. There are many other modalities that address cellulite in a very aggressive — and often painful — manner. They work *into* these micro-adhesions to break them up, and at times this can be a necessary evil to make such work effective. Cups, however, work with negative pressure. Applying them over an area of cellulite should be less about strong suction and more about using the cups skillfully. There is no reason for a painful treatment. Instead, it should feel invigorating or energizing to these stagnant areas.

The total body concept is an important component of treating cellulite. While there may be concentrated areas requiring focus, like the hips and thighs, in this case the entire lymphatic system is sluggish and therefore any treatments should address as much of the body as possible. If nothing more, be sure to address the midsection (torso, glutes and thighs) of the body entirely, as it is the core of lymphatic drainage.

Before you begin applying cups, consider the following:

- The treatment recommended is based on a full body lymphatic drainage, using either moving cups or lift-and-release techniques to both break up areas of stagnation — areas of cellulite — and then systematically flush away fluids that were previously sluggish and congested by the cellulite. This method of application is detailed in Chapter 9, so be sure to have the instructions ready as a guide.
- Use larger cups (relative to body parts) and lubricant, since moving cups are being used. Like lymphatic drainage, larger cups are more effective for the more regional work involved with cellulite. For example, it is more beneficial to address the entire gluteal region with a larger cup than one small cellulite dimple with a small cup because all the *surrounding* tissue is contributing to that one dimple.
- Consider treating the abdomen for constipation before treating the body for cellulite, as this is another contributing factor to a systemic stagnation. (If this is not relevant, feel free to bypass this suggestion.)
- Movements should comfortably follow the contours of the body. This means that when working in the gluteal and hip region, where most cellulite applications will focus, moving the cup in a circular direction is easiest, as it follows the contours of the body. When working on the back of the thighs or upper arms, smaller circles or side-to-side lines of movement (not sliding down the arm toward the elbow, nor leg toward knee — remember how directionally influential cups are with bodily fluids!) can work quite well to break down smaller areas of cellulite. If you cannot work in circles or back and forth in an area — such as the abdomen, where the dermis is thinner and you could potentially irritate the visceral organs — repetitive passes over the area to address lymphatic drainage will also be very effective.

Method of Application

The treatment should start in the lower back and abdominal midsection, then move to the glutes and hips (if self-care, you can reach behind yourself), thighs and upper arms, and end at the upper chest.

The entire body should take less than 30 minutes for treatment.

1. **Increase circulation to any focus cellulite areas.** Apply 5 to 20 (no more) stimulating passes over the area of focus, such as the gluteal region. With light to medium pressure, depending on the person's comfort level, attach the cup to the skin, lift until tension engages and move the cup around the area to create an overall increase in circulation. Remember, while moving cups may be recommended due to their enhanced benefit of separating adhesions as they slide over any tissue, lift-and-release can also be introduced until moving cups are comfortable. This can be a faster, more vigorous application, since you are working to really energize and awaken the sluggish area. Be sure you have plenty of lubrication on the skin so the moving cup slides easily.

Safety Point

Do not overwork any part of the body. Limit the work to 20 stimulating passes. If there is no need to focus on the arms, for example, make only a few draining strokes there to encourage lymphatic drainage. Tissue may be warm and pink — this is a good response but not necessary for optimal benefit.

2. **Immediately follow the lymphatic drainage pathway of that area.** For each area, follow the appropriate lines of movement (from Chapter 9), using lighter suction pressure and either moving or lift-and-release techniques, with a maximum of 5 times but no fewer than 3 times.

   Wherever you are focusing the work (hips, thighs, abdomen), it is imperative that you follow lymphatic drainage pathways *after you have addressed the concentration of cellulite*, because all the stagnant lymph and tissue fluids that were trapped by the cellulite adhesions now need to be drained. If lymphatic drainage is not done afterwards, the work will not be as effective.

3. **Then move on to the next section and repeat the process until finished.** Once you finish addressing the midsection, go on the gluteal region, then continue to the legs, finishing up around the chest and arms. Applications like cupping for cellulite are most beneficial when completed in a logical and methodical manner; therefore, sectional progression over the entire body works best.

Creating a Treatment Plan

This treatment is intense for the entire body system, even though it may not feel like it, so choose two days of the week separated by 48 hours, such as Monday and Thursday or Tuesday and Friday, etc. The time between treatments is necessary for the tissue to fully process the work. Remember that cups create space and influence the movement of fluids. If this work is done every day, you could actually create swelling. So pick one day, let the body process and adjust, then do it again 48 hours later.

Cellulite did not appear in one day, so you cannot get rid of it in one day. There may be some impressive improvements in just one treatment, but pursue the entire process to reap full benefits. Like everything else with cupping, this work is *cumulative.*

PULMONARY CONDITIONS AND CUPPING

The use of cups to treat pulmonary conditions has been popular throughout time. From ancient medical practices to present-day applications, cups can help manage conditions with restricted breathing.

Examples of pulmonary conditions that can benefit include:

- **Asthma** is a condition characterized by chronic inflammation and vasoconstriction (narrowing of vascular bodies).
- **COPD** is a general term used to describe progressive respiratory conditions that are non-reversible. Emphysema, chronic bronchitis and irreversible asthma are just a few conditions that are categorized under this term. The condition is characterized by labored breathing, an inability to take deep breaths or breathlessness, chronic coughing or wheezing and tightness in the chest. COPD is most commonly caused by smoking or long-term exposure to second-hand smoke, as well as prolonged exposure to harmful air pollutants (such as vehicle exhaust) or inhalable substances (such as coal miners inhaling coal dust or agricultural workers inhaling air-distributed pesticides).
- **Bronchitis** is inflammation of the lining of the lungs, which leads to excessive production of mucus that the respiratory system is forced to expel. This can be an acute or a chronic condition. Acute bronchitis is usually the result of an upper respiratory infection and should be resolved once the infection has cleared up. Chronic bronchitis presents the same symptoms but can last a few years. This chronic situation is usually caused by chronic upper respiratory infections, anatomically irregular bronchi, or environmental pollutants, such as cigarette smoke.

CUPPING 101

Hand cupping is taught in various schools of therapy to stimulate the mucociliary action (clearing of phlegm) in the respiratory system. If you don't have cups, try this technique:

Make a "cup" with each of your hands. Picture using your hands to scoop water up for drinking. Apply in a percussive manner (like playing a bongo drum) over the back of the body in the lung region. Be sure to keep the hands cupped so the palms never make contact with the back. Apply these movements quickly and with a light to medium amount of pressure. A minute or so will be beneficial, and perhaps tiring to the one applying the cupping!

• **Coughs and colds:** The average cough that often accompanies a cold is due to some type of upper respiratory infection, which leads to the production of excess mucus that the body is trying to expel by coughing. If choosing to use cups for a cough or cold, make sure that the person is already into the healing phase, so minimally 72 hours after the initial onset of sickness. The more severe the sickness, the longer you should wait to apply cups during recovery.

• **Shallow breathing:** Many physical and emotional factors can contribute to breathing with limited capacity. Postural distortions such as scoliosis can cause labored or shallow breathing. These distortions in turn affect the diaphragm, the intercostal muscles contained within the rib cage and all accessory breathing muscles, limiting their capacity for full movement. Emotionally stressed individuals (with depression, for example) tend to have very limited, labored breathing, which can have negative effects on the entire breathing mechanism if it persists. Continuous shallow breathing can manifest physically as neck and shoulder pain, for example, if the accessory muscles become overworked.

There are many other pulmonary conditions that can also benefit — evaluate the particular condition you may want to treat with cupping and approach accordingly.

Method(s) of Application

Flash cupping is a more traditional application of cups and yields significant results for pulmonary congestion. This method mimics hand cupping — a percussive form of a *tapotement*, which is like drumming with the edge of your hand or fingertips.

To do this with cups, you will need multiple cups and some dexterity. It requires applying and removing cups more quickly than most applications, over and over the same general region of the body. Flash cupping will work best on the back of the body, between the shoulder blades and along both sides of the spine, directly over the rib cage (and underlying lung tissue).

To do this:

▸ Apply cups all over the lung region (rib cage and between shoulder blades). Suction pressure can vary according to the person's comfort.

▸ Since this is a faster application, allow cups to remain in place for a minimum of 10 seconds but no longer than 1 minute. Apply, remove, reapply.

This vigorous application is intended to stimulate the mucociliary escalator (the combined efforts of mucous and cilia within the respiratory system that trap and remove unwelcome substances from the area) of the lungs to help loosen and remove the deeply embedded phlegm.

For Pulmonary Conditions

STATIONARY CUPS OR FLASH CUPPING, PRONE POSITION

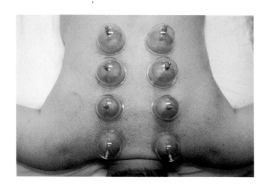

Manual cups have been used for demonstration. Apply cups over the lungs from the back of the body. Applications can be stationary here (to facilitate deeper releases, such as drawing out inflammation associated with asthma) or flash cupping can be used in the same positioning for a more stimulating and productive application.

- Begin placing cups in between the shoulder blades, in the upper back.
- Place cups one at a time, along either side of the spine.
- The bottommost cups should be placed above the bottom line of the rib cage, about one hand's width above the back hip bones.
- For flash cupping, remove and replace cups repeatedly in the same locations.
- For a stationary, deeper application (like addressing asthma), allow cups to remain in place for a maximum of 3 minutes but no less than a minimum of 30 seconds.
- Whichever application is used, remove cups in the order they were applied for the best relief.

STATIONARY CUPS, SUPINE POSITION

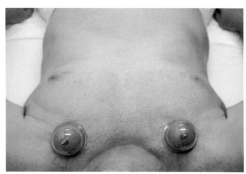

Place one cup over the pectoralis minor muscle, on each side of the upper chest. Placing cups directly over this location addresses both this accessory breathing muscle, as well as powerful lung-stimulating points used in other alternative therapies.

- To find these placement points, use your fingertips to locate the clavicle (collarbone). Starting from the center of the chest, slide your finger along the length of it until you reach a soft indentation; this is the area where the pectoralis minor muscle is attached to the acromioclavicular (AC) joint.
- Place the cup in the soft space just below the AC joint, approximately 2 to 3 fingers' width below the collarbone.
- Allow the cups to remain for a maximum of 3 minutes, but no less than a minimum of 30 seconds. Remove cups one at a time.

MOVING CUPS, PRONE POSITION

Moving cups stimulate overall circulation to all the muscles and tissue surrounding the lungs. Apply moving cups to the back of the body, covering the entire rib cage region.

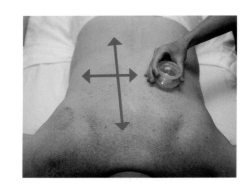

Rib cage: Sliding a cup over the entire rib cage greatly benefits pulmonary conditions. Considering the natural tightness of the diaphragm and intercostals, located within the ribs, this application alone provides instant relief.

Move the cup all along the contours of the available rib cage space. The shoulder blades cover a portion of the rib cage, so if a moving cup can comfortably be used over them (but don't scrape the cup on the shoulder blade), then it will add to the overall application.

▸ Apply a good amount of lubricant to the skin so the cup slides easily.
▸ Address one side of the body entirely first, then the other.
▸ Starting up between the shoulder blades along either side of the spine, attach a cup with a light to medium suction pressure.
▸ First direction: Begin sliding the cup up and down alongside the spine. The bottommost point should be before the end of the rib cage, and the topmost point should be at the top of the shoulder, below where the neck meets the shoulder.
▸ Second direction: Begin sliding the cup across the width of the rib cage, below the shoulder blade, from alongside the spine and out toward the sides of the body, ending at the person's side body. If needed, mark a line straight down from their armpit to mark an endpoint. Slide the cup back and forth here; this space is short, sliding the cup around the rib cage just below the shoulder blade, and ending above the bottom of the rib cage.

PREGNANCY AND CUPPING

Massage and bodywork are a welcome relief from the aches and pains a mother-to-be will experience as her body shifts and changes over the course of her pregnancy. Some of the most common physical discomforts associated with pregnancy include restricted muscle and fascia along the back and hips, as well as swelling in the face, hands and feet. There can also be a lot of emotional stress during this time, and some simple therapeutic cupping can be gently infused into any massage and bodywork session to help bring some much-needed comfort. Cupping can also complement other bodywork by moving stagnant fluids and creating space in tighter areas without irritating the mother-to-be's body, which may be hypersensitive during this time.

Safety Point

As with any application, if you are unsure whether someone can receive cupping — or bodywork — during pregnancy, be sure to check with their doctor before attempting it.

Though therapeutic cupping can be a valuable tool during pregnancy, keep in mind these factors and considerations.

- **Cups are contraindicated during the first trimester.** This is the time when the body is making decisions, building and stabilizing. Bodywork is typically contraindicated during the first trimester unless the pregnant mother has been receiving regular bodywork from a trained professional.
- **During pregnancy, there is an increase in blood volume and fluids.** Therefore, lighter suction must be used because there is a greater tendency to bruise or create more swelling.
- **While it is normal to have some swelling (particularly in advanced pregnancy), an excess of swelling can be extremely dangerous.** If pitting edema occurs (an indentation remains after gently pressing a fingertip into the skin), this could mean that the kidneys are unable to filter blood and toxins and immediate medical attention is required, and absolutely no cupping or bodywork.
- **Blood clots can occur in the legs during pregnancy.** As a consequence, any cupping work should be done with only the lightest lymphatic intentions.
- **The sensory receptors in the body can be altered by the changes in skin and levels of bodily fluids.** This change results in hypersensitivity of the skin and muscle tissues, so be sure to monitor how the recipient is feeling while working on the body, with or without cups.

Rules of Cupping during Pregnancy

- **Little to no cupping in the midsection of the body.** The lower back, sacrum, pelvis and around the entire abdomen are locations that require the utmost protection and safeguards.
  - *Cups work to release adhered tissue*, and in this region of the body the baby *needs* all the adhesions created to ensure proper security and support.
  - *Cups work to move fluids.* Again, the baby *needs* the fluid in this region to remain where it is. Using cups in the midsection could throw off the delicate balance the body is maintaining.
  - *Cups can lift and stretch tissues wherever applied.* During pregnancy a special hormone (relaxin) is produced that allows ligaments and muscles to relax and stretch to allow the baby to move down into proper positioning. After childbirth, this hormone is no longer produced and the body works to bring back the tonicity of such ligaments and muscles. Any added stretch with cups could potentially cause lasting damage.
- **Absolutely *no* cups in the *abdomen*, ever.**
- **In general, use only the lift-and-release technique.** Considering the fluctuation in the levels of bodily fluids and the power of moving cups to shift fluids in a literal wave of movement, moving cups may be too powerful for the body to process. Stationary cups — practically *anywhere* on the body — could also be too powerful for the body during this time. Instead, use *only* lift-and-release technique, especially if you are attempting to alleviate some swelling in the arms and legs.

Basic applications and techniques not to use during pregnancy:

- **Cups for constipation.**
- **Cups for acid reflux.**
- **Cups directly over the lower back region,** including lower back muscles, lumbar spine, sacrum and pelvic bones. Considering all the attachments the body has created for the baby, as well as the altered state of tissue, do not use cups here, to avoid any damage. Massage is safe and welcomed during pregnancy because massage techniques press in, while cups lift and separate.
- **Stationary cups on the limbs.** The arms and legs tend to retain fluids, so any stationary applications may only contribute to this issue.
- **Cups along the inside of the legs and around ankles or feet.** There are powerful elimination points along the foot, around the ankles and all along the inside of the legs all the way up to the groin.
- **Cups for pulmonary conditions**, as the areas treated are too close to the midsection.

Why Use Cups during Pregnancy?

There *are* some effective applications for muscle work or gentle fluid movements during pregnancy, though cups need to be applied safely and with less intensity.

- **Cups for stress relief:** During this period of volatile emotions, any soothing and stress-relieving treatments are welcome. Relaxing applications along the upper back, neck and shoulder can stimulate the parasympathetic nervous system, thereby triggering the release of relaxing neurotransmitters, which systematically offers relief to the entire pregnant body. Lift-and-release technique works very well here, or a gentle moving cup can be used over the upper shoulder region.

- **Cups for sciatica:** Cups can effectively relieve sciatica discomforts; however, pay attention to the location of cupping. For example, do not use cups over the lumbar spine, sacrum or along the pelvis; rather, use cups in the center of gluteal muscles or closer to the hip joint. Using the lift-and-release technique, think of these applications as spot-treating where muscles may be tighter.

- **Cups for neck and shoulder tension:** Cups are safest to use up in the neck and shoulders. Just remember not to be too aggressive or strong with the work, and no cupping below the shoulder blades.

- **Cups for the limbs:** While moving cups of any suction pressure would move too much fluid, the arms and legs respond well to the gentle application of cups with light suction pressure and the rhythmic application of the lift-and-release technique. Such an application aids in improving overall circulation and fluid retention in the limbs that may occur during pregnancy.

  - When addressing limbs, remember to treat a proximal area (upper thigh, upper arm) before treating a distal area (lower legs, lower arms). See Chapter 9 for more information.

  - Always work toward the torso when treating limbs. Again, a cup can move fluid anywhere you guide it, so working down an arm or leg can only increase the swelling. Also, working toward the torso supports the natural direction of veins, while working in the opposite direction could potentially cause vascular damage (such as varicose veins).

Cupping during this time is quite limiting and limited. It should be. Most of the body is focused on one thing: the baby. Cups exert a full systemic influence and should be minimal for the duration of the pregnancy.

Safety Point

Remember, there is also a tendency for blood clots in the limbs during pregnancy, so be sure the work is light and the intention is to address the lymphatic system.

SCAR TISSUE AND CUPPING

DID YOU KNOW?

Scars can also form from burns, acne, chicken pox and other conditions that affect the layers of the skin.

There are various types of scar tissue, both internal and external. When soft tissues rebuild from even the smallest injury, scar tissue forms and remains in the body. Any cuts into the skin (surgical, injury, etc.) immediately cause scarring, creating external, visible scar tissue. Internal scar tissue can occur in a variety of ways, such as when muscles are damaged, fascia is restricted or visceral organs fail to function properly. The good news is that all scar tissue responds positively to cupping.

By nature, scar tissue has a different composition due to its atypical formation during the repair process. When tissue is damaged, the body rebuilds it with newer, thicker and stronger tissue fibers very similar to the previously existing tissue. When these two tissues combine, however, the newly formed irregularity can lead to restrictions often associated with scar tissue.

This section will deal specifically with scars that form when the tissue is cut: atrophic, or "regular," and hypertrophic, or "atypical," scars (including keloid scarring; see more information on this type of atypical scarring later in the chapter). How scars heal can be influenced by several contributing factors:

- The severity of tissue damage (size or depth of injury)
- The location on the body (face versus leg tissue)
- The direction of damage (does it go with or against the tissue fibers, 'the grain'?)
- Local blood supply (e.g., poor circulation)
- Medications and how they might affect the tissue repair process (e.g., steroids, birth control pills)
- Type of tissue, color or density (light or dark skin pigment, foot or abdominal tissue)
- Age of skin (youth or senior citizen)

Atrophic Scars

Atrophic scars are caused by cuts to the skin. Regardless of how deeply the cut penetrates, these scars are generally even with the surface of the skin or slightly sunken. As the damaged tissue is being repaired, new and altered collagen fibers and connective tissues begin to grow, parallel to the surface tissue. The deeper the cut (surgery versus soft tissue injury), the more complicated the atrophic scarring may be. As the scar forms, it may become augmented from the connective tissue that is helping to rebuild the area and its ever-changing anatomy, potentially creating adhesions or thicker areas of the scar. The more complicated or restricted the scar, the more involved the local anatomy can become. Some surface scars can lead to deeper fascial and muscular adhesions, potentially limiting function and range of motion. Deeper scars (surgical) can sometimes create adhesions that affect visceral organs, nerves and bones.

Cupping with Atrophic Scars

Scars have responded quite well to massage techniques like friction and myofascial release. Such manipulations press into the tissue, however, whereas cups lift the tissue without pressing on an already compressed area. Cupping is very disorganizing to the cellular matrix of the newly formed connective tissues and can draw blood into — and encourage fluid to move through —whatever tissue is bound within the scar itself. Laceration scars can often trap blood and perhaps foreign debris (for example, glass from a motor vehicle accident) within the newly formed tissue layers and lead to further restrictions. The body works very hard not only to expel these unwelcome materials, but also to stabilize and strengthen the damaged area. Cupping lifts, separates and decompresses these tissues; the potential for release and promoting healthy tissue is very high.

THERAPEUTIC THOUGHT: SCAR TREATMENT

From my experience, individuals who receive scar work often remark that they feel a considerable difference within the scar tissue. I always suggest that they feel the scar with their fingers first — the texture, the sensations, the surrounding area. Then I treat the scar with cups and ask them to feel the scar again. I haven't met anyone who did not feel a positive change. From a quick lift-and-release application to a longer, detailed treatment, scars respond very well to cupping. The biggest challenge, however, is making sure to not overwork the tissue. Remember, any work done with cups is cumulative.

New Scar Tissue versus Old Scars

NEW SCARS

The newer the scar, the more gently you must work tissue. Adding this style of therapeutic cupping into the recovery process may improve the health of the new tissue as well as potentially reduce the visible scarring. *Caution should be exercised with newly forming scars:* Never use cups if there are any scabs, stitches, adhesive materials or new, raw skin present. If the tissue is not completely and thoroughly healed before applying this therapeutic work, you run the risk of reopening the scar. Since you are working with new collagen fibers and connective tissues, cupping that is too strong can overstimulate the production of such fibers and contribute to the irregularity of scar tissue rather than soften it. Cupping can also help alleviate the inflammation that accompanies the formation of new scar tissue (see "Working with Inflammation," page 224 for more information).

Do not begin cupping on scar tissue until approximately 6 weeks after the tissue was cut. If the tissue seems more compromised, wait longer. If you're unsure, ask for medical approval for scar massage before proceeding.

CUPPING 101

For an introductory general application, choose a cup that is considerably larger than the width of the scar to address all the surrounding tissue as well as the scar line. This allows for dispersed suction over the entire area and helps to assess how the skin will react. There is surrounding tissue to consider when attempting this work.

OLD SCARS

The older the scar, the more strongly you can work tissue. While visible results may not be as dramatic as with new scars, the potential for visible change still exists, as does improving the internal composition and overall texture. Cupping helps disorganize the excessive binding and restrictions that accompany scars — imagine the amount of restriction that may be involved. The decompressive nature of cups can relieve pressure on any anatomy around the scar, including muscles, nerves and organs. All of this promotes healthier tissue in the region, softening and releasing binding patterns that may have been limiting local function or comfort. Remember that this work is cumulative, so start with basic applications, and if there is a desire to lengthen the time of work or intensity of cupping, do so with the person's comfort in mind.

Cups also allow fluids — both blood and lymph — to move through previously obstructed structures on older scars, bringing about the potential for some significant changes to these challenged areas. Picture a dam in a river, and how it stops water moving along its path and causes it to swell around the dam, altering the landscape. Now compare this to a scar and what it can do to the circulation of blood, the movement of lymph and the anatomy around it.

Cups and Newer Atrophic Scar Tissue

Using cups with newly forming scar tissue is meant to be light and work in conjunction with the body's natural rebuilding processes. Be sure that it has been *approximately 6 weeks* since the tissue was cut before attempting any work. Below is a step-by-step application for newly forming scar tissue.

For New Atrophic Scar Tissue

LIFT-AND-RELEASE OR MOVING CUPS, SUPINE POSITION

With newer scars, encourage some lymphatic drainage before you begin. Such an application will stimulate the lymphatic system for what is to come, as well as support its natural function during this time of heightened activity. Inflammatory responses may make addressing lymphatic movement soon after any surgical procedure too sensitive, so be mindful and work according to the recipient's comfort level.

There is no need for stationary cups over new scars, since this would draw too much fluid into the area. The light, softening and fluid-moving treatment with lift-and-release or moving cups is beneficial for new scar tissue — it helps promote softer, more hydrated and "normal" tissue formation during this period of reconstruction.

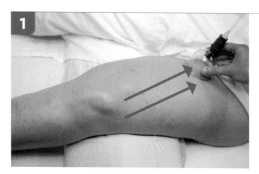

1 Encourage lymphatic drainage by using the lift-and-release technique or gentle moving cups with light suction pressure. In this example, I worked above the knee, upwards along the thigh and inward toward the groin and femoral triangle region, where inguinal lymph nodes are located.

For step-by-step instructions and directions on addressing lymph movement and drainage, see Chapter 9: "Therapeutic Cupping for Lymphatic Drainage"; this example is Step 12 of the full body drainage for the front of the thigh, page 211.

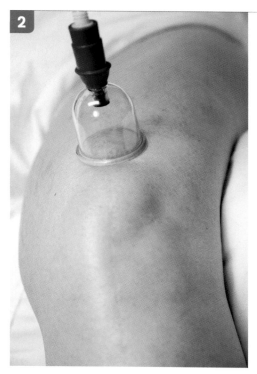

2 Treat the entire scar directly. For newer scars, use the lift-and-release technique for initial applications (2 or 3 sessions), then you may choose to use moving cups with *very* light suction pressure along the length of the scar if desired. The more compromised the tissue, the longer you should use only the lift-and-release application so the tissue is not being lifted and separated too much. Remember, moving cups have a wave-like effect on the tissue as they slide along, and even the lightest moving cup can be too much for some people if applied too soon. Test the area a little before proceeding.

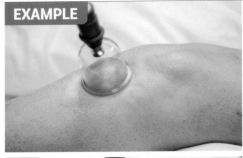

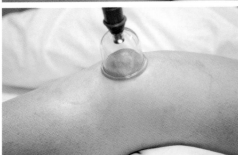

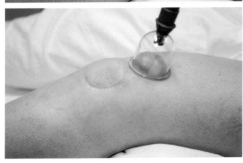

In this example, the scar is from a knee replacement surgery, and it runs lengthwise over the knee joint and lower thigh. The leg is supported by a pillow; be sure whatever body part you are working on is fully relaxed and supported, if necessary.

- Place the cup directly over the scar, locating the scar line in the center of the cup to the best of your ability.
- Begin by applying the cup along the entire length of the scar line.
- In this example, I began working at the bottom of the scar, then progressed upwards to the top of the scar. If the scar runs across the body or in some other direction (diagonal, crooked scar line), begin at one end of the scar line and progress along the entire length of it, one cup width at a time. Optimally, begin at the most distal point and work your way in, but with some scars (like cesarean section scars) this is not possible. Instead, be sure to simply address the entire length of the scar, and then follow appropriate direction of lymphatic drainage pathways thereafter. For example, with a cesarean-section (c-section) scar, you would work down through it, toward the inguinal lymph nodes located in the groin area.
- Whatever direction is appropriate, progress along the length of the scar, using either technique (lift-and-release or a moving cup).
- Remember to attach the cup *lightly*. Use a very light tension, especially for new scar tissue cupping.
- Repeat this line of movement (along the length of the scar) for a maximum of 5 times but no less than 3 times.

Note

Notice the lymphatic fluid coming into the tissue, where the previous cup placements were applied (above, bottom picture).

Repeat Step 1 after directly treating the entire scar to continue lymphatic movements.

The entire treatment should take about 15 minutes but no less than 5 minutes. The larger the scar or the more sensitive the area, the more time may be needed.

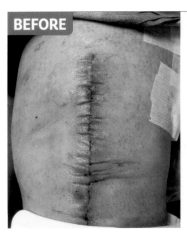

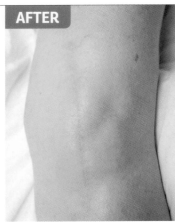

BEFORE: This picture was taken a few days after knee replacement surgery. We waited 2 months before starting any cupping applications due to a complicated recovery.

AFTER: This photograph was taken 8 months after the surgical procedure. Treatments were done twice weekly, for 5 consecutive weeks (10 sessions), then once a week for 6 more weeks, and then every other week for 2 more months. In total, 5 months of regular applications.

C-Section Scar

The first photo shows a scar 8 weeks after a C-section, before the first cupping application. Because it was a new scar, the applications began with light lift-and-release applications over the entire scar and along the lymphatic drainage pathways for 4 initial sessions, done twice weekly for 2 weeks. Light moving cups were introduced for the following 4 sessions (twice weekly for 2 weeks), and then we added the application of stationary cups directly over the scar line for another 4 sessions (twice weekly for 2 weeks). After that, sporadic visits (every few months) included stationary cups and moving cups all over the scar line and general area. The second photo was 1 year later, when she was pregnant again.

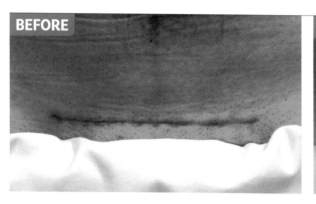
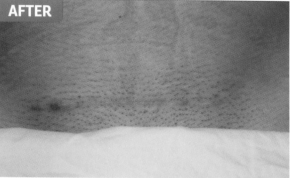

BEFORE

AFTER

Hypertrophic and Keloid Scars

Scars that grow beyond their own borders are known as hypertrophic or keloid scars. Hypertrophic scars stay within the line of the scar but rise above the surrounding surface tissue. Keloid scars can grow above the skin surface as well as extend beyond the borders of the scar, sometimes growing into irregular forms. Both scars form as the result of an excessive production of collagen, usually from an infection during the healing phase.

Cupping with Hypertrophic and Keloid Scars

Working with these volatile scars should be done only by trained professionals with advanced knowledge of such delicate and complicated scar tissue. Given how cups can increase tissue activity (increase circulation, stimulate nerve endings), any aggressive cupping could worsen the scar. Strong cupping might awaken the body's healing response and trick it into thinking that the scar is being irritated, thereby triggering it to produce even more collagen.

References

ARTICLES

Athletic Performance

Young sub Kwon, MS and Kravitz L, PhD. How do muscles grow? *IDEA Fitness Journal*, 2006 Feb; 23–25. Available at: http://www.ideafit.com/fitness-expert/young-sub-kwon.

Applications

Fairclough J, Hayashi K, Toumi H, Lyons L, Bydder G, Phillips N, Best TM, Benjamin M. The functional anatomy of the iliotibial band during flexion and extension of the knee: implications for understanding iliotibial band syndrome, J Anat. 2006 Mar; 208(3); 309–316. Available at: www.ncbi.nlm.nih.gov/pmc/articles/PMC2100245/.

Kenny T, as reviewed by Imm N. Heel and foot pain (plantar fasciitis), Doc. 4311 (v42) Last checked 2/2/16. Available at: https://patient.info/health/heel-and-foot-pain-plantar-fasciitis.

National Institute of Neurological Disorders and Stroke. Carpal tunnel syndrome fact sheet, 2017 Jan. Available at: www.ninds.nih.gov/Disorders/Patient-Caregiver-Education/Fact-Sheets/Carpal-Tunnel-Syndrome-Fact-Sheet.

Body Systems

Turchaninov R. How massage therapy heals the body. Part III: vasodilation mechanisms, 2011 Jul. Available at: https://www.scienceofmassage.com/2011/07/how-massage-therapy-heals-the-body-part-iii-vasodilation-mechanisms/#.

Cupping Marks

Bentley B. A cupping mark is not a bruise, *The Lantern*, Vol 12–2. 2015.

Edema

Chris DR. Edema (swelling) and anasarca (generalized body swelling), www.healthhype.com. Available at: http://www.healthhype.com/what-is-edema-body-swelling-pathophysiology-causes-types.html.

Emotions

Pert, CB. The wisdom of the receptors: neuropeptides, the emotions, and bodymind. Advances 3: 8-16, 1986, 8–16.

Face Lymphatic Drainage

Shannon A. Techniques for face lifting and drainage using vacuum micro-cups, TheraCupping LLC, 2011, Asheville, NC.

Fibromyalgia

Weiss J. Breakthrough in fibromyalgia research: pain is in your skin, not in your head. *Medical Daily*, 2013 Jun. Available at: http://www.medicaldaily.com/breakthrough-fibromyalgia-research-pain-your-skin-not-your-head-246925.

General Reference

Mehta P, Dhapte V. Cupping therapy: a prudent remedy for a plethora of medical ailments, J Tradit Complement Med. 2015 Jul; 5(3): 127–134. Published online 2015 Feb 10. Available at: https:www.ncbi.nlm.nih.gov/pmc/articles/PMC4488563/.

Rozenfeld E, Kalichman L. New is the well-forgotten old: the use of dry cupping in musculoskeletal medicine. J Bodyw Mov Ther. 2016 Jan;20(1):173-8. doi: 10.1016/j.jbmt.2015.11.009. Epub 2015 Dec 1.

History

Bentley B. Explorations of cupping in Greece, *The Lantern* Vol 10–1. 2013.

Inflammation

Butterfield TA. Best TM, Merrick MA, The dual roles of neutrophils and macrophages in inflammation: a critical balance between tissue damage and repair, J Athl Train. 2006 Oct–Dec; 41(4): 457–465. Available at: https://www.ncbi.nlm.nih.gov/pmc/articles/PMC1748424/.

Nordqvist C. Inflammation: chronic and acute, *Medical News Today*, last updated Wed 16 Sept 2015. Available at: http://www.medicalnewstoday.com/articles/248423.php.

pH information

Kulkarni AC. Kuppusamy P, Parinandi N, Oxygen, the lead actor in the pathophysiologic drama: enactment of the trinity of normoxia, hypoxia, and hyperoxia in disease and therapy, *Antioxidants & Redox Signaling*, Oct 2007, 9(10), 1717–1730. Available at: https://doi.org/10.1089/ars.2007.1724.

Schwalfenberg GK. The alkaline diet: is there evidence that an alkaline ph diet benefits health? Journal of Environmental and Public Health, 2012 J Environ Public Health. 2012; 2012: 727630. Published online 2011 Oct 12. doi: 10.1155/2012/727630.

Pulmonary

Rushton L. Occupational causes of chronic obstructive pulmonary disorders, Rev Environ Health. 2007 Jul-Sep;22(3):195-212. Available at: www.ncbi.nlm.nih.gov/pubmed/18078004.

BOOKS

Barnes JF. *Myofascial Release, the Search for Excellence*. A Comprehensive Evaluatory and Treatment Approach. 10th ed. Pennsylvania, PA: Rehabilitation Services, Inc.; 1990.

Chirali I. *Traditional Chinese Medicine Cupping Therapy*. 2nd ed. Edinburgh, UK: Churchill Livingstone Elsevier; 2007.

Edmonson JM. *American Surgical Instruments: An Illustrated History of their Manufacture and a Directory of Instrument Makers to 1900*. San Francisco, CA: Norman Publishing; 1997.

Földi M, Ströbenreuther R. *Foundations of Manual Lymph Drainage*, 3rd ed. St. Louis: Elsevier Mosby; 2004.

Guimberteau JC, Armstrong, C. *Architecture of Human Living Fascia. The Extracellular Matrix and Cells Revealed Through Endoscopy*. Williston, VT: Handspring Publishing Ltd.; 2015.

Korthuis RJ. *Skeletal Muscle Circulation*. San Rafael, CA: Morgan & Claypool Publishers; 2011.

Mapleson T. *A Treatise on the Art of Cupping: In Which the History of that Operation Is Traced, the Complaints In Which It Is Useful Indicated, And the Most Approved Method of Performing It Described*. Princes Street Soho: London Wilson; 1830.

Meyers TW. *Anatomy Trains. Myofascial Meridians for Manual & Movement Therapists*. 3rd ed. Edinburgh, UK: Churchill Livingstone Elsevier; 2014.

Pert, CB. *Molecules of Emotion: The Science behind Mind-Body Medicine*. New York, NY: Simon & Schuster;1999.

Pittman RN. *Regulation of Tissue Oxygenation*. San Rafael, CA: Morgan & Claypool Life Sciences; 2011.

Purves D. *Neuroscience*, 2nd edition, Sunderland, MA: Sinauer Associates; 2001.

Salvo, SG. *Massage Therapy Principles and Practice*. Philadelphia, PA: W.B. Saunders Company; 1999.

Upledger, J. *Somato Emotional Release and Beyond*. Palm Beach Gardens, FL: Upledger Institute; 1990.

WEBSITES

Crystalinks, Metaphysics and Science, www.crystalinks.com/egyptmedicine.html (Egyptian history)

Greek Medicine.net, www.greekmedicine.net (Greek history)

Hijama Nation Academy, www.hijamanation.com (Islamic culture)

National Center for Biotechnology Information, www.ncbi.nlm.nih.gov

Sports Injury Clinic, www.sportsinjuryclinic.net/sport-injuries/shoulder-pain/frozen-shoulder (Frozen shoulder)

RESOURCES (CUPS)

Carbo Medical Supplies
www.carbo.ca, (800) 370-9077

Electro-Therapeutic Devices, Inc. (ETD)
www.etdinc.ca, (877) 475-8344

Shannon Gilmartin
www.moderncuppingtherapy.com

Acknowledgments

Thank you to my loving family.

To my father, Tom, for always believing in me and guiding me along the road of life. Love you, Dad.

To my loving mother, Jackie, for being the greatest mother and friend every step of the way, along with being a grammatical genius!

To my brother, Jason, for being the bestest big brother, mentor and voice of reason a sister could ever have.

To my beautiful nephews, Jacob & Evan and Ethan, for playing along with your silly aunty, and thank you to the most excellent Gilmartin and Leiby families for a lifetime of love and support.

Thanks to all those who have supported me along the way, personally and professionally: Paula F. Gilmartin, Marie Melia, Deena Taddia, Momma Linda and the Sheehan-Black family, Jen, Mandy Pannone, Stacie Nevelus, Miryah Nielsen, Mariliz Vega Anderson, Tanisha Balarezo, 'Sista' Vickie Thompson, Stephanie Wheatley, Susan Sandage, Mark Pawley, Megin Kennitt, Kassy Klein, Scott and Eliza Cohen, Khadija, Joel Ganz, Cynthia Lewis, and Dr. Rich.

A special dedication to my late stepfather, Sal, and in loving memory of Sweet Melissa.

Sincerest gratitude to Brenda Brown, Rob Watson and all the wonderful teachers who have helped to shape my therapeutic mind over the years, and to all my clients and students for giving me the opportunity to cultivate my body of work throughout my career.

Thank you to my willing subjects who donated their time to make the photography of this book possible: Megin K., Amy Y., Marilliz A., Alyssa S., George C., Mark P., Donna and Jerry, Debbie P., Vickie T., Joel G., John K., Gina G., Kent T. and Mom.

Thank you to Anita Shannon for introducing me to the wonderful world of cups and for encouraging my own personal growth and development within the field of vacuum therapies. A special thank you to my business partner, the lovely Stacie Nevelus. Also, thank you to the effervescent Randy Heaps, Beth-Ellen Zang, William Burton and Annie Garic.

Thank you to Bob Dees at Robert Rose Publishing for giving me this incredible opportunity, as well as Marian Jarkovich and Martine Quibell for their marketing and publicity efforts, Fina Scroppo for her phenomenal (and patient) editing, and Kevin Cockburn and the team at PageWave Graphics Inc. for their exceptional design work. Thank you to Sze-Linn Choong and Kevin Liu with ETD and Carbo Medical Supplies, Tammy Leiner of the Longevity Centers of America for providing the thermographic images, Dan Wunderlich and all the volunteers of Global Healthworks Foundation, and photographers Douglas James (for my headshot) and Jennifer Steele (for the book photography).

I'd like to also acknowledge contributions by Stacie Nevelus, 'Sista' Vickie Thompson and Susan Sandage, D.Ac.

To all family and friends around the world who have contributed in some way to help bring me to this point, thank you.

Library and Archives Canada Cataloguing in Publication

Gilmartin, Shannon, 1979-, author
    The guide to modern cupping therapy : your step-by-step source for vacuum therapy / Shannon Gilmartin, CMT.

Includes index.
ISBN 978-0-7788-0583-0 (softcover)

    1. Cupping. 2. Cupping — Handbooks, manuals, etc. 3. Cupping — Popular works. I. Title.

RM184.G55 2017   615.8'9   C2017-905234-9

Index